Martin Stolz

Functional analysis across dimensions: from tissues to atoms

AF062664

Martin Stolz

Functional analysis across dimensions: from tissues to atoms

Diagnostics at the nanoscale

Südwestdeutscher Verlag für Hochschulschriften

Impressum/Imprint (nur für Deutschland/only for Germany)
Bibliografische Information der Deutschen Nationalbibliothek: Die Deutsche Nationalbibliothek verzeichnet diese Publikation in der Deutschen Nationalbibliografie; detaillierte bibliografische Daten sind im Internet über http://dnb.d-nb.de abrufbar.

Alle in diesem Buch genannten Marken und Produktnamen unterliegen warenzeichen-, marken- oder patentrechtlichem Schutz bzw. sind Warenzeichen oder eingetragene Warenzeichen der jeweiligen Inhaber. Die Wiedergabe von Marken, Produktnamen, Gebrauchsnamen, Handelsnamen, Warenbezeichnungen u.s.w. in diesem Werk berechtigt auch ohne besondere Kennzeichnung nicht zu der Annahme, dass solche Namen im Sinne der Warenzeichen- und Markenschutzgesetzgebung als frei zu betrachten wären und daher von jedermann benutzt werden dürften.

Coverbild: www.ingimage.com

Verlag: Südwestdeutscher Verlag für Hochschulschriften GmbH & Co. KG
Dudweiler Landstr. 99, 66123 Saarbrücken, Deutschland
Telefon +49 681 37 20 271-1, Telefax +49 681 37 20 271-0
Email: info@svh-verlag.de

Approved by: Basel, University, Dissertation, 2002

Herstellung in Deutschland:
Schaltungsdienst Lange o.H.G., Berlin
Books on Demand GmbH, Norderstedt
Reha GmbH, Saarbrücken
Amazon Distribution GmbH, Leipzig
ISBN: 978-3-8381-2975-4

Imprint (only for USA, GB)
Bibliographic information published by the Deutsche Nationalbibliothek: The Deutsche Nationalbibliothek lists this publication in the Deutsche Nationalbibliografie; detailed bibliographic data are available in the Internet at http://dnb.d-nb.de.

Any brand names and product names mentioned in this book are subject to trademark, brand or patent protection and are trademarks or registered trademarks of their respective holders. The use of brand names, product names, common names, trade names, product descriptions etc. even without a particular marking in this works is in no way to be construed to mean that such names may be regarded as unrestricted in respect of trademark and brand protection legislation and could thus be used by anyone.

Cover image: www.ingimage.com

Publisher: Südwestdeutscher Verlag für Hochschulschriften GmbH & Co. KG
Dudweiler Landstr. 99, 66123 Saarbrücken, Germany
Phone +49 681 37 20 271-1, Fax +49 681 37 20 271-0
Email: info@svh-verlag.de

Printed in the U.S.A.
Printed in the U.K. by (see last page)
ISBN: 978-3-8381-2975-4

Copyright © 2011 by the author and Südwestdeutscher Verlag für Hochschulschriften GmbH & Co. KG and licensors
All rights reserved. Saarbrücken 2011

Contents of Thesis

1.	**General introduction**	8
2.	**Thesis overview**	11
2.1	Systematic study of biological matter at all levels: From bones to atoms	12
2.1.1	The asymmetric unit membrane (AUM) – a model membrane for the investigation of the urothelical plaque formation	13
2.1.2	Imaging actin arrays at molecular detail on positively charged supported lipid layers	13
2.1.3	Elasticity measurements of soft biological tissues	14
2.2	Instrumentation The methodical armamentarium of structural biology	15
2.2.1	Light microscopy (LM)	16
2.2.2	Transmission electron microscopy (TEM)	17
2.2.3	X-ray crystallography	18
2.2.4	Nuclear magnetic resonance (NMR) spectroscopy	20
2.2.5	Scanning probe microscopy (SPM)	20
2.2.5.1	AFM used in this thesis	21
2.2.5.1.1	Contact-Mode AFM	23
2.2.5.1.2	Tapping-Mode AFM	23
2.2.5.1.3	Force-Mapping (FM) AFM / Indentation-Type (IT) AFM	24
2.2.5.2	Sample preparation for AFM for imaging in physiological environment	25
2.2.5.3	Immobilization strategies of biological matter for high resolution AFM	26
2.2.5.4	Examples	27
2.2.5.4.1	"Spontaneous" adsorption of amyloid-like fibrils	27
2.2.5.4.2	Adsorption of 2D membranes by electrostatic balancing	28
2.2.5.4.3	Adsorption of actin arrays by adjusting the appropriate surface charge	28
2.2.5.4.4	Transfer of 2D protein crystals onto hydrophobic surfaces by the monolayer method	29
2.2.5.4.5	Binding of biomolecules to solid supports by silanization	29
2.2.5.4.6	Preparing articular cartilage for AFM imaging	30
2.2.5.4.7	Preparation articular cartilage for elasticity measurements	31
2.2.5.5	Imaging biological specimens by AFM	32
2.3	References	33

3	Imaging the luminal and cytoplasmic face of the asymmetric unit membrane (AUM) by AFM in their functional state	39
3.1	Introduction	39
3.2	Materials and Methods	40
3.2.1	Materials	40
3.2.2	Isolation and negative staining of AUM plaques	40
3.2.3	Atomic force microscopy	41
3.3	Results and Discussion	43
3.3.1	Height measurements of the AUM	43
3.3.2	Visualization of fully native urothelial plaques by AFM	43
3.3.3	Comparison of AFM with negative stain EM and cryo-EM	46
3.3.4	Structural features of the 16-nm plaque particles as obtained by cryo-EM, negative stain EM and AFM	48
3.3.5	Visualization of dynamic processes: from "snap shots" to movies	50
3.3.5.1	Temporal resolution of dynamic biological processes at the molecular scale	50
3.3.5.2	Integrated and indirect methods for time-resolved studies	51
3.3.5.3	Direct assessment of time-resolved mechanistic processes at the level of single molecules by microscopic techniques	51
3.3.5.4	Observation of the putative rearrangement of urothelial plaque particles while bladder distention by using time-lapse AFM	52
3.3.6	Conformational changes might occur and triggered by chemical or mechanical effectors	53
3.4	Conclusion	54
3.5	References	55
4	AFM of native actin polymers and crystals after stable immobilization on supported lipid bilayers	59
4.1	Introduction	59
4.2	Materials and Methods:	61
4.2.1	Materials	61
4.2.2	Actin	61
4.2.2.1	Preparation of actin	61
4.2.2.2	Preparation of F-actin paracrystals	62
4.2.2.3	Preparation of crystalline actin sheets and tubes	62
4.2.3	Atomic force microscopy	62
4.2.4	Electron Microscopy	63
4.2.5	Immobilization of disperse F-actin filaments and of paracrystalline arrays of actin filaments on charged lipid monolayers starting with G-actin	63
4.2.6	Immobilization of actin sheets and tubes on synthetic charged supported lipid bilayers	65
4.3	Results and Discussion	67
4.4	Conclusions	72

5	**Assessing the biomechanical properties of normal, diseased and engineered tissue by indentation-type AFM**	**77**
5.1	Assessing the mechanical properties of porcine cartilage tissue at the nanometer and micrometer scale by indentation-type AFM	78
5.2	Relevance of elasticity measurements of articular cartilage tissue by indentation-type AFM	79
5.2.1	Methods used for characterization of mechanical properties	80
5.2.1.1	Hardness	80
5.2.1.2	Elastic modulus	82
5.2.1.3	Indentation testing device resolution capability	83
5.2.1.4	Corollaries	84
5.3	Dynamic elastic modulus of articular cartilage determined at two different levels of tissue organization by indentation-type AFM	85
5.4	Introduction	86
5.5	Materials and methods	89
5.6	Results	94
5.7	Discussion	102
5.8	Conclusions	111
5.9	Other potential applications in biology, medicine and bioengineering	112
5.9.1	Quality control of engineered tissue or biomaterials	112
5.9.2	Exploring the vulnerability of coronary artery plaques	114
5.6	References	116
6	**Summary and outlook**	**121**
6.1	There is no such thing like an ideal microscope	121
6.2	Further developments in instrumentation	123
6.2.1	Probes	124
6.2.2	Putative applications of AFM-based techniques in medicine	126
6.3	References	127

1. General Introduction

1 General introduction

In 1959 Richard Feynman, the Nobel Laureate physicist, gave a visionary lecture[1] entitled "There is plenty of room at the bottom". This speech stimulated his audience with the vision of opportunities for nanotechnology. How small, he wondered, could machines be built? He finally concluded, "The principles of physics, as far as I can see, do not speak against the possibility of maneuvering things atom by atom". In the same talk he referred to Albert R. Hibbs, who suggested a very interesting possibility for fabricating relatively small machines. He said that, although it is a very wild idea, it would be interesting in surgery if you could swallow the surgeon. You put the mechanical surgeon inside the blood vessel and it goes into the heart and "looks" around. This now famous speech of Richard Feynman is generally attributed as the birth of nanotechnology.

About twenty years later, the technique of scanning tunneling microscopy (STM; (Binnig, et al., 1982)) provided the "eyes" and "fingers" required to measure and manipulate matter at the atomic and molecular level. In 1986, the invention of the atomic force microscope (AFM; (Binnig, et al., 1986)) broadened the technology to non-conductive surfaces and especially to the world of living matter.

If it was just the length scale involved in the definition of the prefix "nano" then nanotechnology and nanoscience could be considered to have been around for decades. However it is clearly not that simple. The tremendous advances in microelectronics and computer industry that are based on manufacturing electronic devices smaller, faster and cheaper might be a good example for approaching the world of the nanometer scale. However, at the same time the use of this top down approach reveals the limits of the current technology. At the so-called quantum-limit, i.e. at the scale below ~20 nanometers, the conventional laws of physics change and new rules apply. Therefore it is not enough to scale down our daily experience of reality how we perceive it from our perch in space-time. New non-orthodox concepts going beyond the framework of classic principles will provide us with new insights and a new way of looking at, understanding and interpreting nano-scale phenomena. Moreover, it is essential to develop the ability to work at these levels with the perspective to generate larger structures with a fundamentally new molecular organization.

---

[1] This classic talk was given by Richard Feynman on December 29th 1959 at the annual meeting of the American Physical Society at the California Institute of Technology (Caltech).

One of the most exciting aspects of nanotechnology might be related to the rational or *de novo* construction of nanomachines (Gimzewski, *et al.*, 1998; Gimzewski, *et al.*, 1997). To this end, biological systems demonstrate how organic molecules in living organisms assemble themselves into complex supramolecular structures exhibiting distinct functionalities: The rotary flagellar motor that propels bacteria or the actin-myosin system that powers muscle, represent two examples from the living world that demonstrate that molecular machines do indeed exist and function. Nanotechnology seeks to understand how they work and to build them for technological use.

2. Introduction to the Thesis

2 Thesis overview

A significant amount of nanoscale research is underway around the world – the United States, Japan, Western Europe, and many other countries – that might eventually lead to dramatic changes in the ways that materials, devices, and systems are understood and created. To this end, a variety of national programs are supporting long-term nanoscale research, to advance our understanding of the underlying principles and mechanisms governing living matter that ranges from the study of the structure and dynamics of biomolecules, such as proteins and nucleic acids, all the way to cells, organs and organisms. Nanotechnology is intimately associated with biology because all living systems are governed by the behavior of atoms and molecules at the nanoscale. Therefore nanotechnology can provide us with new innovative routes for probing the world of the living matter, and hence, may result in new analytical tools that could have a profound impact on structure research, medicine and health care. At the same time, it may stimulate the refinement of preparation protocols for imaging, measuring and manipulating biomolecules, organelles, cells and tissues.

In this context, structure research of living matter is the key to eventually correlating the molecular architecture of biological systems with their functions. However, successful and efficient study of a biological system strongly depends on asking the right biological question, choosing an appropriate method, and optimally preparing the specimen so as to maintain its structural and functional integrity. To provide a detailed answer to a biological question modern structural biology involves a variety of fundamentally techniques to investigate the biological matter of interest. However, the complexity of the biological specimen in terms of size and shape, consistency (multiphasic systems) and localization of the biomolecule, whether isolated or representing an integral part of the biological tissue, and consequently the requirements in terms of resolution and functionality, reduce the choice of available tools. Well frankly spoken most of today's tools in fundamental science and surgery are simply too large to examine and manipulate with structures at our level of interest.

The first part of this thesis describes the biological matter at its different levels of organization, i.e. tissue, cells, organelles, membranes, supramolecular assemblies, biomolecules and atoms. This is followed by an overview of the state-of-the-art microscopical techniques and novel capabilities for complementing the "integrated methodical approach" presently used in the life sciences. Next, I am presenting three different types of applications that are of considerable interest in the biomedical sciences. I'm introducing the AFM as a member of the family of scanning probe microscopes followed by the specific way it was used for these studies, which includes the preparation protocols of each of the individual biological samples. My primary goal is to demonstrate the relevance of AFM-based techniques with these three examples that are described in detail in the main part of this thesis. Last but not least, I want to give an outlook to some difficulties that remain to be resolved, in terms of sample preparation and instrumentation, as well as summarizing some recent developments in instrumentation and putative applications of the methods discussed in this context for science and health.

2.1 Systematic study of biological matter at all levels: From bones to atoms[2]:

As the telescope enables us to catch a glimpse of the universe, computerized X-ray tomography and magnetic resonance imaging (MRI) allow us to look inside our body and image its skeleton and organs in three dimensions. Similarly, with the microscope we can explore the microcosmos, from cells and tissues all the way down to molecules and atoms. For example, by "cutting" optical sections the confocal laser-scanning microscope (CLSM) allows us to look inside living cells and tissues, and to resolve their cytoskeleton and various organelles. Using video-enhanced light microscopy, cell structures can be visualized whose dimensions is one order of magnitude or more below the resolution limit of the light microscope and has enabled molecular motors to be directly observed at work. The electron microscope (EM) can cover an even wider range of dimensions from imaging whole cells, their organelles, the cytoskeleton and supramolecular assemblies, as well as individual biomolecules, their submolecular structure and, ultimately, individual atoms. However, to withstand the high vacuum inside the EM, biological specimens have to be dehydrated thus causing them to denature and become subject to preparation artifacts. One way out of this dilemma has been the introduction of liquid nitrogen – or even liquid helium-cooled cold stages to preserve the specimen in a thin film of amorphous ice while inspected or imaged in the EM. Another attempt to keep biomolecules in their native environment has been to embed them in glucose syrup. However, due to the low inherent contrast of biological matter when embedded in ice or glucose, only crystalline specimens (e.g., 2-dimensional (2D) crystalline protein arrays or icosahedral virus capsids) can be imaged at high resolution by these two methods. Recently, the atomic force microscope (AFM) has opened completely new vistas for analyzing the surface topography of biological matter in its aqueous environment at a resolution comparable to that achieved by EM. Most exciting, the AFM is the first imaging device allowing direct correlation between structural and functional states of biomolecules at submolecular resolution.

[2] **M.E. Müller Institue for Microscopy booklet, From bones to atoms, second edition 1996**

2.1.1 The asymmetric unit membrane (AUM) - a model membrane for the investigation of the urothelical plaque formation

As a first example, we succeeded to image the luminal and cytoplasmic faces of the asymmetric unit membrane (AUM). The AUM forms numerous "plaques" covering the apical surface of the mammalian urinary bladder epithelium. Each plaque consists of 16 nm-sized diameter protein particles that are hexagonally packed (Kachar et al. 1999; Walz et al. 1995). We performed AFM of completely native AUM plaques with the goal in mind to eventually construct a 3D model depicting the structural organization of individual plaque particles. Further on we want to understand how adjacent plaques are held together by "hinges" and how distinct plaques and hinges are forming. Another prospect is to investigate the plaque particles in response to various chemical and physical effectors that might interfere with its natural functioning in the human bladder. Moreover, the AUM plays a fundamental role in bladder infection, where E. coli bacteria adhere onto the plaque particles as the first step in this pathogenesis (Min et al. 2002; Wu et al. 1996). However, the mechanism as well as the precise docking site has to be better understood. To achieve these goals, a protocol had to be developed to obtain stable adsorption of both faces of AUM plaques.

2.1.2 Imaging actin arrays at molecular detail on positively charged supported lipid layers

As a second example, we set out to prepare various types of actin arrays for high resolution AFM imaging with the longer-term goal in mind to eventually watch individual myosin motors stepping along actin filaments. Actin exhibits a myriad of diverse functions, most of which ultimately depend on its intrinsic ability to rapidly assemble and disassemble filamentous structures (Schoenenberger et al. 1999). Actin controls the mechanical stability of the cytoskeleton and thereby the overall shape and motility of cells. Actin is also directly involved in muscle contraction were actin filaments (F-actin) are serving as "molecular tracks" for myosin motors to step along. Kinesins and dyneins are other motor proteins that specifically interact with microtubules. In this latter case the two-headed motor protein kinesin moves along microtubule tracks in a linear fashion. Myosins, kinesins and dyneins convert chemical energy derived from adenosine triphosphate (ATP) hydrolysis to mechanical force (DiBella and King 2001; Shih et al. 2000; Vale and Milligan 2000). Upon ATP hydrolysis the actin-based motor protein myosin generates mechanical force by a large conformational change, i.e. the so-called power stroke, in a cyclic manner as do kinesins and dyneins. Kinesins and dyneins are molecular motors that develop speeds at the order of hundreds of nm/sec and forces on the order of several piconewtons (Mogilner et al. 2001).

Hence, the cyclic chemo-mechanical force generation by these molecular motors forms the molecular basis of biological motion, by this in the form of muscle contraction, cell motility, or the vectorial transport of cargoes along molecular tracks, and by that a fundamental aspect of life (Schoenenberger and Hoh 1994). In this context AFM potentially offers the possibility to watch muscle contraction at work with molecular resolution, i.e. to trace myosin heads with an SPM tip in their different conformational states during their cyclic interactions with actin filaments. To eventually achieve this ambitious goal, we have been trying to image F-actin filaments but also G-actin arrays under native conditions by AFM, not only to compare the native structure of the filament with its atomic model, but also to eventually directly monitor structural changes induced by chemical or mechanical effectors. To this end, I have been able to achieve the stable immobilization of various G- and F-actin arrays in physiological buffers.

2.1.3 Elasticity measurements of soft biological tissues

As a third example, we used the AFM for *ex vivo* measurements of cartilage elasticity as taken under physiological buffer conditions. The elastic modulus of cartilage is a material parameter that directly relates to the absorption and transduction of forces through joints and thereby combines structural data of the cartilage architecture with information obtained by biochemical analysis (Cohen et al. 1998; Franz et al. 2001; Hayes et al. 1972; Jurvelin et al. 2000; Shepherd and Seedhom 1997; Tkaczuk 1986). For providing a robust reference database, an automated method was developed, that we refer to as indentation-type (IT) AFM, for directly computing the dynamic elastic moduli from the load-indentation curves provided by the AFM, or by employing a calibration standard using agarose gels with known elasticity. Next, dynamic elastic moduli at two different scales, i.e. at the nanometer and at the micrometer scale were determined for different cartilage tissues such as native, diseased, enzymatically treated or engineered articular cartilage.

Elasticity measurements of articular cartilage using cantilevers with attached spherical tips with a diameter of ~5 μm were in accordance with published values, whereas nanoelasticity measurements performed by sharp, nm-sized tips revealed values that were typically 100-fold lower. Enzymatical digestion on articular cartilage that specifically degraded distinct components of the tissue, i.e. proteoglycans (PGs), glycsoaminoglycans

(GAGs) or the collagen moiety, allowed us to correlate microindentation data (i.e. measured by spherical tips) to the overall tissue elasticity (Bader and Kempson 1994; Bader et al. 1992), whereas elasticity values obtained by nanoindentation testing (i.e. measured by sharp nanometer-sized tips) could therefore be related to the PG and GAG content of the cartilage's extracellular matrix (ECM)

For a more practical and medical relevant application, the sensitivity of our method might enable us to use the dynamic elastic modulus, especially the provided nanoelasticity, as a sensitive and thus early indicator of cartilage malfunction (osteoarthritis) (Kaab et al. 2000; McDevitt and Muir 1976; Roth and Mow 1980), or as a parameter of quality control for tissue-engineered cartilage (Vunjak-Novakovic et al. 1999). In the case of those synthetic cartilage engineered in bioreactors the potential application will be in replacing damaged tissues in patients with impaired cartilage function due to acute (e.g. trauma) or chronic (e.g. osteoarthritis) tissue damage (Langer and Vacanti 1993; Peppas and Langer 1994). Ultimately, we also want to develop these AFM-based elasticity measurements into a clinical tool yielding diagnostic information, for example, by putting an AFM-based device into an arthroscope for direct *in situ* diagnosis by minimally invasive procedures on biomechanics of hydrated soft tissues, for example, an AFM-based device for *in vivo* arthroscopic surgery (Appleyard et al. 2001; Aspden et al. 1991; Dashefsky 1987).

2.2 Instrumentation: The methodical armamentarium of structural biology

Complementary structural information about biological specimens can be obtained by using crystallographical, spectroscopical and microscopical techniques. Most of the structural data available is produced by light microscopy (LM) including confocal microscopy, electron microscopy (EM), X-ray crystallography and nuclear magnetic resonance (NMR) spectroscopy. X-ray crystallography provides atomical structures, NMR-spectroscopy yields information on the chemistry of biomolecules and electron microscopy localizes the site of the specimen in the cell and visualizes the overall organization within the tissue.

Spectroscopic approaches, i.e. X-ray diffraction and NMR spectroscopy yield primary data that are difficult to directly interpret. For most of us "seeing is believing" because the human mind can quickly grasp spatial relationships when presented in pictorial form, and consequently a micrograph might be worth "a thousand words" or columns upon columns of spectroscopical data.

The primary advantage of microscopes are three-fold: (i) they directly produce images rather than diffraction patterns or spectras; (ii) they enable us to explore biological structures at all levels from the macroscopic to the atomic scale; and (iii) they allow biological matter to be imaged in its functional environment (Stoffler et al. 1999).

To explore the structure and function of proteins and their supramolecular assemblies by microscopes, a range of different instruments are available that depending on the exact nature of the specimen and the structural information seeked, may be employed individually or in combination by an integrated methodical approach.

2.2.1 Light microscopy (LM)

Light microscopy (LM), i.e. polarizing, interference, fluorescence and confocal microscopy all allow observation of the specimen in physiological buffer environment. For LM the sample often does not need any special treatment or preparation and the operation of these instruments is relatively easy and straightforward. This is definitely one reason why LM-based techniques are most popular in biology. With computer-aided video-enhanced LM the tracking of motion and cellular dynamics can directly be followed even on a subsecond time scale.

In a conventional LM the magnified image of an object is produced by a series of glass lenses. According to E. Abbé the diffraction limited resolution is directly dependent on the wavelength of the light used. Hence the practical resolution achieved in an LM is about 200 nm thus preventing a detailed analysis of fundamental processes of life that take place on a smaller scale. Nevertheless LM has been an extremely valuable tool for biologists over the past fifty years. It is typically used to gain structural and dynamical information of biological matter from the tissue or whole cell level, to the cytoskeleton and distinct organelles. In addition, it is well suited to track motion of entire cells, distinct cellular compartments and organelles and has been used to look at motions on the surface and the interior of the cell. Unfortunately due to its relatively low resolution a detailed insight into the more molecular details of cellular processes are not possible, at least not in a routine fashion.

2.2.2 Transmission electron microscopy (TEM)

Transmission electron cryo-microscopy (cryo-EM) is a valuable tool for detailed structural investigation of specimen structures that are embedded in a layer of vitrified ice. From a series of 2D projections of particles with proper alignment, a 3D structure can be reconstructed. A prominent example for this is the hepatitis B capsid protein, which adsorbs and orients in a random fashion onto the grid (Henderson and Unwin 1975; Mancini et al. 1997; Unwin and Henderson 1975). By classification of the macromolecular faces, alignment of the images and backprojection exploiting the high symmetry of the virus, a reconstruction of the 3D structure was determined with a resolution sufficient to visualize the secondary structure, i.e. it was possible to identify individual α-helices (R.A. Crowther, MRC, Cambridge). For larger and irregular macromolecular assemblies such as chromosomes, viruses and organelles cryo-electron tomography offers to study the 3D ultrastructure using a tilt stage to record a series of projection images at different angles (Grimm et al. 1998; Voges et al. 1994).

The instrument based resolution power of a modern EM is at best of about 1Å. Typical structures investigated by EM are often larger than those investigated by X-ray crystallography or NMR. Most samples of material sciences applications like minerals or metals tolerate a higher dose of electrons and therefore can be imaged at a high signal-to-noise ratio that is the prerequisite for atomical resolution. In contrast, the resolution for biological specimens can be significant lower, because the electron exposure for biomolecules must be as low as 5 e/Å^2 to avoid resolution loss by radiation damage. As a consequence, the individual EM image suffers from a poor signal-to-noise ratio. To date, only crystalline specimens (e.g., 2D crystalline protein arrays) allow the reconstruction of an atomical model computational by image processing exploiting the crystalinity of the sample. Moreover, cryo-specimen preparation of protein molecules, protein complexes, and cell organelles embedded in vitrified ice requires a high degree of technical skill to prevent disruption of macromolecular arrangements. Existing high-dose cellular tomography only yields macromolecular resolution.

The resulting images are digitized, and must be aligned with respect to one another and averaged to reduce noise for an interpretable restoration of the structure. Obviously, the attainable resolution will critically depend on the accuracy of alignment, which, in turn, depends on the signal-to-noise ratio of the individual images. This alignment problem can best be solved with periodic specimens, for example 2D crystals, helical polymers or icosahedral virus shells, which due to the structural redundancy present in the crystalline particles provide a "rule" for aligning the repeating units relative to one another (Opalka et al. 2000).

Beside the high price for a state-of-the-art instrumentation, the major drawback concerning EM in biology is that EM techniques can only provide "snap shots" of the biological specimens "immobilized" in a thick layer of vitrified ice. By freezing the sample after triggering a reaction or the start of a cycle, time-resolved snapshots of up to 5 msec accuracy can be obtained (Ruiz et al. 1994). EM is able to visualize the structures of motor proteins and their tracks, i.e. actin and myosin (Amos et al. 1982; Schroder et al. 1993), tubulin and kinesin at (near) atomic resolution as well as the motor decorated filaments (Hoenger et al. 1995), but it is inherently not able to trace the cross bridge cycle of actin decorated actin filaments, kinesin-decorated microtubles or to follow movements and shape changes that are fundamental processes of biological matter and life. Another application of cryo electron tomography is to provide a context for the localisation of biomolecules and subcomplexes within a cell, a ribosome or a virus. In this way components of known atomic structure determined by either X-ray crystallography or NMR can be fitted as rigid bodies into EM maps of larger macromolecular complexes.

2.2.3 X-ray crystallography

X-ray crystallography is not an imaging but a spectroscopic technique that uses 3D crystals as specimens to determine macromolecular structures of proteins. There is a number of protein structures available that is solved to ultrahigh resolution (better than 1.0 Å) and most atomic structures of proteins, i.e. over 80% of the three-dimensional macromolecular structures in the Protein Data Bank have been determined by X-ray crystallography.

When an X-ray beam passes through a crystal the lattice serves as a diffraction pattern to scatter the electromagnetic radiation. Depending on the arrangement of atoms in the molecule an array of diffraction peaks or Bragg reflections is recorded on a X-ray detector. Depending on the crystal order, X-ray crystallography readily yields atomic detail of the asymmetric unit representing the basic building block of the crystal. Higher resolution results in a more accurate determination of atomic positions.

However, to obtain the accurate molecular structure good quality crystals of the molecule must first be obtained. So far, many important molecules failed to produce suitable crystals. As yet, only for tubulin that can be packed into highly ordered 2D crystals (i.e. the Zn sheets), the resolution was good enough to eventually yield an atomic model. For actin, myosin and kinesin the attainable resolution has been much worse. All those examples were provided by electron crystallography instead of X-ray crystallography.

Once a crystal is obtained the raw data, i.e. a diffraction pattern of thousands of spots can be produced. From a technical point of view the phase problem has to be solved, that means that the diffraction pattern registers only the intensity of the waves and the phase information must be mathematically obtained either from the diffraction data or experimentally determined from supplementing diffraction experiments. By the so-called "direct method" (Richardson and Jacobson 1987; Salisbury et al. 1997; Sheldrick et al. 1978), a mathematical approach for molecules smaller than $\sim 10^3$ (1000) non-hydrogen atoms, the phases are evaluated from the measured diffraction intensities by using relationships among the phases based on a priori knowledge about crystal structures like atomicity and non-negativity of the electron density distribution. For larger molecules another method is normally used, called "isomorphous replacement", which is based on the insertion of heavy metal atoms into the crystal structure. Apart from direct methods and MIR (Guss et al. 1988; Hendrickson 1991), molecular replacement can be used to phase diffraction data from molecules of size. Molecular replacement (Chothia and Lesk 1986; Chothia et al. 1986) generates initial phases by the correct placement of a structure from a known homologue into the crystal lattice of the unknown structure. An initial phase estimate can be obtained from such a model if its orientation in the crystal lattice can be determined.

In contrast to X-ray crystallography EM-diffraction of 2D crystalline specimens allows recording the phase information. Therefore, both techniques can be used as complementary tools. However, it has been only in very few cases where cryo-EM and X-ray crystallography have been combined. Examples are the low-resolution structure of ribosomes and icosahedral viruses. In those two examples higher resolution X-ray crystallography data revealing the structures of the subcomponents and those are combined with the lower resolution "overall" structure obtained by cryoEM that provide a context for these structures by showing their spatial arrangement. Thioredoxin from E. coli is another prominent example for a molecule that has been studied in complementary methods of structural biology, namely by X-ray crystallography and by solution NMR (see Protein Data Bank, http://www.rcsb.org).

One limitation of X-ray crystallography is that no direct information about the molecule's dynamic behavior is available from a single diffraction experiment – again, all you get are "snap shots", as of EM.

2.2.4 Nuclear magnetic resonance (NMR) spectroscopy

Nuclear magnetic resonance (NMR) spectroscopy detects resonances of nuclei and gives a spectrum of peaks that reveals detailed structural information. In a strong magnetic field some nuclei ($1H$, $15N$, $13C$, ...) exhibit characteristic splitting of energy levels of nuclear spins. Their magnetic moments subsequently orient themselves parallel or anti-parallel to the magnetic field. By applying an alternating radiofrequency field transitions between these different nuclear spin states can be induced (Ernst et al. 1987).

The molecular composition and chemical bonds of an individual protein results into a characteristic electron density distribution and to a slightly different magnetic field at the sites of the nuclei relative to their isolated state. NMR spectroscopy is sensitive to those small changes that the nuclei experience in a protein. Frequency transitions are induced at slightly different resonances in a NMR spectrum, which can be measured directly.

The resulting spectra can be analyzed in conjunction with various other techniques, e.g. mass spectrometry, infrared spectroscopy and Raman spectroscopy to determine the complete structures of proteins in solution or of an unknown compound. Mass spectrometry is used for the determination of the size of a molecule and its molecular composition, infrared- and Raman spectroscopy for the identification of some functional groups present in a molecule. To date, high resolution NMR is typically restricted to molecules of a molecular weight of up to 50 kD and is therefore of little use to determine the atomic structure or to study conformational changes of large biomolecules.

For clinical applications, the related magnetic resonance imaging (MRI) is frequently used as a diagnostic technique for *in vivo* tissue imaging that produces high quality images of the inside of the human body. However, magnetic resonance imaging lacks detailed structural information at the level of living cells or smaller because at the present time its spatial resolution is limited to about 1 mm (Rubenstein et al. 1997; Sinclair et al. 1982).

2.2.5 Scanning probe microscopy (SPM)

In 1981 Gerd Binnig and Heinrich Rohrer invented the scanning tunneling microscope (STM) for which they received the Physics Nobel Prize in 1986, a clear manifestation of its significance (Binnig and Rohrer 1982). The STM allowed for the first time to directly image material surfaces at atomic detail. The operation of an STM is based on the so-called tunneling current, which starts to flow when a sharp metal tip approaches a conducting surface at a distance of approximately one nanometer. Another breakthrough came in 1986 with the introduction of the atomic force microscope (AFM) by Binnig, Quate and Gerber (Binnig et al. 1986). The AFM allows the observation of surface topography of non-conductive samples at the atomic level. Hence, the AFM appeared very suitable for looking at biological material.

Today, STM and AFM are the parents of a wide range of scanning probe microscopes (SPMs), that all exhibit a common feature: a sharp, tiny probe that approaches the sample surface to a few Å to monitor a physical parameter of the specimen while the sensor is scanned line by line over the specimen surface. The feedback from the sensor is used to keep the strength of the interaction (current, force, amplitude,...) constant, so that a constant probe signal is maintained (Miles 1997). Most SPMs can be operated in air, vacuum, but also in liquid, including electrolytes.

There are three main modes of AFM operation that are currently in use: contact, non-contact and intermittent mode. As yet a "real" non-contact mode has not been developed for the usage in liquid. In tapping or intermittent contact mode the cantilever is oscillated near its resonance frequency while operating in the repulsive force region. In order to reduce damage to potentially fragile samples, i.e. biological matter, the surface is touched only for short periods of time. In addition, the force-mapping mode (FM AFM) and the pulsed force mode (PF AFM) (Miyatani et al. 1997) enable high-resolution mapping of adhesion, stiffness, elasticity and energy dissipation. In those measurements the scanning tip is placed over the sample surface and then the sample is pushed against the tip thereby producing local indentation into the specimen. The materials information can be obtained from the applied load versus distance curve between probing tip and sample.

2.2.5.1 AFM used in this thesis

AFM is an imaging technique that is fundamentally different from traditional microscopes, because it does not employ any lenses to create an image. Instead, a sharp stylus at the end of a long cantilever contours the object as the tip scans over the sample. In high resolution imaging the force between tip and sample is kept constant and at minimal interaction with as little as much deformation. The AFM senses the sample surface height as a function of position producing a quantitative 3-dimensional map of the surface. One key feature is the extremely precise lateral and vertical displacement capability of the sharp probe tip relative to the sample surface by a computer-controlled piezo scanner that allows accurate measurements of heights and distances.

In contrast to EM and X-ray crystallography AFM does not need quick-freezing, fixing, embedding, and staining of the specimen for faithful preservation of its details. AFM data have a high signal-to-noise ratio that does usually not require signal averaging for contrast enhancement.

In a light microscope the resolution limit is imposed by the wavelength of visible light, in an EM the resolution is increased by using electrons instead of photons and for an AFM the resolution is given by the sharpness of the probe. When directly comparing EM and AFM, as two microscopical methods that cover about the same range of resolution, the AFM often provides a slightly smaller resolution than obtained by EM. However, the AFM often offers enough resolution to trace the relevant changes of small particles, filamentous assemblies and planar structures such as membranes and two-dimensional (2D) protein crystals. Sometimes it might be very useful, or even the only way, to combine different techniques.

Next, I want to give an example for an integrated approach that allows to answer biological questions by combining LM, EM, X-ray crystallography, NMR and scanning probe microscopies, i.e. to investigate structural and functional aspects of biomolecules: The nuclear pore complexes (NPCs) are large macromolecular assemblies of 120 MDa with an overall diameter of 120 nm and an overall height of roughly about 100 nm. These huge molecular machines are embedded in the double membrane envelope of eukaryotic cells where their major functioning is to mediate the molecular trafficking of ions, small molecules, proteins, RNAs, and ribonucleoprotein particles between the nucleus and the cytoplasm. This bidirectional molecular transport between the cytoplasm and the cell nucleus is fundamental for the proper functioning of the cell. So far, it has not been possible to crystallize NPCs into a lipid membrane for making them available for the EM followed by offline image processing where the averaging of a large number of unit cells could eventually allow obtaining an atomic model. However, in structure-based approaches the building blocks of the NPC, for example, the NLS binding domains or nucleoporins are currently under investigation by X-ray analysis. Once a high resolution 3D structure is determined by X-ray analysis, Cryo-EM-tomography can then be used to fit some of these sub-complexes within the NPC. In this context, AFM does not yet offer a resolution as obtained by EM or X-ray analysis, but it has sufficient resolution to study effector-specific conformational changes, correlating with the functional dynamics of the NPC as it relates to nucleocytoplasmic transport.

Moreover the NPC is a good example for both, EM and AFM, that in most cases it is not the instrument but the nature of the specimen that limits the attainable resolution. However, the biological question is the primary goal and the obtainable resolution provided by the combination of technique and specimen is only one special aspect for the choice of a specific technique.

AFM also allows monitoring the growth of macromolecular crystals, following the assembly of complexes between RNA polymerase and DNA, and depicting conformational changes directly and in physiological buffer environment. For an understanding of molecular machines, the motor proteins and their tracks can be assessed independently in their different conformational states, and the mechanism can be directly traced in space and time, something that might be only monitored or visualized by employing an AFM.

AFM-based mechanical testing is a novel application in this field that potentially allows for a complete mechanistic understanding at different levels of biological tissue organization, i.e. of the structural organization and related functioning from the single-molecule level to the complex interaction of the entangled interaction of all building blocks. The AFM's ability to image, measure, manipulate and organize biomolecules on the nanometer scale is of great significance in fundamental research as well as in many applications in the life sciences. Of particular importance is the potential use of the AFM in clinical applications, for example, for early detection diagnosis and therapeutic interventions of symptoms before diseases become apparent.

Next, I want to give a brief overview about the different scanning modes that were relevant for my doctoral thesis, i.e. contact-mode AFM (CM AFM), tapping-mode AFM (TM AFM) and force-mapping AFM (FM AFM).

2.2.5.1.1 Contact-Mode AFM

When highest resolution of protein molecules to be imaged in aqueous buffer solution is required contact-mode AFM (CM AFM) is the operational method of choice. A prerequisite for achieving highest resolution with soft biological material is stable immobilization of the specimen on a solid support while kept in buffer solution. In CM AFM the stylus is always in contact with the sample surface and therefore a maximum sensitivity for smallest structural inhomogenities is provided.

2.2.5.1.2 Tapping-Mode AFM

Many biological samples can not be sufficiently stably immobilized on a solid support, or they are too soft or "spongy" to withstand the lateral forces applied to them via the tip CM AFM. In many cases better results in terms of resolution are often achieved by so-called tapping mode atomic force microscopy (TM AFM) (Hansma et al. 1995; Putman et al. 1994). In tapping mode the cantilever is driven at or near its resonance frequency and interactions between the tip and the specimen is sensed by changes in the amplitude of the oscillating tip that gets damped when it barely hits or "taps" the sample while the tip is scanned over the specimen. TM AFM enables observation of molecules without running the risk of the sample being swept or moved away during scanning by a drifting setpoint such as commonly experienced with CM AFM. In TM AFM the lateral or friction forces are drastically reduced because the sample is only physically touched for a short time by the tip when at the lowest position during its oscillation cycle. Therefore TM AFM minimizes lateral forces so that weakly adsorbed single molecules might still be imaged, which eventually might not be possible in CM AFM. In general, the resolution as obtained on the same sample with TM AFM is slightly lower than that in CM AFM (Moller et al. 1999).

However, when employing TM AFM a better resolution can be achieved due to a proper immobilization onto the supporting surface that was achieved by optimization of the surface charge. From that point further improvement of resolution was achieved by a lateral stabilization of filaments by assembling them into loosely packed paracrystalline arrays of filaments. So far, the best spatial resolution on actin oligomers could be achieved on well-ordered 2D crystalline arrays of actin sheets.

In TM AFM the damping of the free amplitude is kept constant by the instrument. Hence, TM AFM is the imaging mode of choice for recording growth processes of real-time monitoring at a longer time scales up to several hours. A prominent example is time-lapse AFM of amyloid fiber growth adsorbed onto mica by time-lapse AFM, where the growth of filaments is followed over time scales up to several hours (Goldsbury et al. 1999; Stolz et al. 2000).

2.2.5.1.3 Force-Mapping (FM) AFM/ Indentation-Type (IT) AFM

In addition to imaging, the AFM can also be used to measure micro- and nanomechanical properties of biological specimens, for example (visco-) elasticity or rupture forces of single molecules at high spatial and force resolution. By employing the force-mapping mode of an AFM the tip is scanned laterally over the sample surface while continuously recording force curves pixel by pixel. At each sample point the sample is pushed against the tip, while recording (i) the Z-displacement of the piezo tube and (ii) the bending of the cantilever (i.e. by an optical detection system) up to a maximum deflection which is set by a trigger threshold. The optical detector system is recording the bending of the cantilever up to a force difference of typically 10 pN. Such AFM-based nanoindentation readily allows monitoring a 0.01 nm displacement resolution (in Z-direction), typically corresponding to forces up to 10 - 50 pN (Engel et al. 1999; Shao et al. 1996). As an example that will be discussed later in this thesis, such nano- and microindentation testing do yield mechanical properties of the specimen such as its hardness or its elastic modulus. Importantly, the apparent stiffness or elasticity of biological tissues such as bone or cartilage will strongly depend on the probe size, i.e. it can differ by several orders of magnitudes depending on the scale of investigation.

As documented later on this thesis I started to develop and scrutinize an AFM-based approach (Stolz et al. 1999) to image cartilage and measure its stiffness. Since our method required several changes to the established indentation testing as developed in the material sciences we refer to our method as indentation-type AFM (IT AFM).

2.2.5.2 Sample preparation for AFM for imaging in physiological environment

As already indicated above a prerequisite to eventually succeed in performing high resolution AFM of large biomolecular assemblies or the characterization of functional aspects of biological tissue is the stable immobilization of the sample on a solid support without compromising its native functional properties and behavior. Since specimens can easily deteriorate during preparation or inspection, protocols have to be developed for maintaining the integrity of the biological structure upon immobilization (Hegner et al. 1993; Karrasch et al. 1994; Wagner 1998; Wagner et al. 1996; Wagner et al. 1994). The first step in sample preparation for AFM is the choice of the "right" substrate. The major requirements for a suitable support and the proper adhesion of the specimen in regard to biofunctionality are as follows:

- Ideally, high resolution AFM imaging requires an atomically flat and biological inert supporting surface to which the biological specimen is attached in a nondestructive but yet stable way.

- Nondestructive imaging that maintains the integrity of a soft specimen requires application of a minimal force between tip and sample surface, especially if structure-function relationships of the native biological material want to be depicted. This, in turn calls for optimizing the imaging mode, i.e. contact versus tapping mode, but it also rely upon refining the image conditions mainly in terms of the ionic strength and pH of the buffer.

- For nanoindentation testing the surface should be as flat a possible so that a controlled and reproducible specimen interaction between the probe and the sample surface is achieved. Moreover the specimen should be thick enough so that its surface properties are not influenced by the underlying solid support.

- Immobilization of the specimens on a solid support must be stable, yet the chemistry of the adhesive or glue should not alter the structural and/ or functional properties of the specimen.

2.2.5.3 Immobilization of biological matter for high resolution AFM: Alteration of the specimen support (i) in terms of its charge or hydrophobicity (ii) by chemical functionalization, and (iii) by coating it via LB-films or self-assembled monolayers

Most of the commonly used specimen supports are charged in an aqueous environment and so are biological specimens. A number of biological membranes and supramolecular assemblies adhere strongly and stably to mica and hence this support is most commonly used with biological specimens. Mica is a mineral that is characterized by a layered crystal structure so that cleavage yields an atomically flat, negatively charged surface. Moreover for most biological specimens mica represents a biological inert surface that is atomically flat over several square micrometers. However, the exert biomolecules and biomolecular assemblies that do not stably adsorb to mica and hence other immobilization strategies have to be explored.

One way to immobilize biomolecules to a solid support is by appropriate chemical modification of the supporting surface. For example, this can be achieved by coating the support with a functional reagent so that it can chemically react with the specimen surface. Hence, by systematically varying the choice of the reactive head group a biofunctional reagent while leaving this tail group an affected one and the same solid support can be customized for many different specimens. In this notation the head group of the biofunctional reagent and the tail group of the supporting surface.

The crosslinking layer coating the specimen support surface must not be necessarily just one layer thick but it can be multilayered thereby involving several preparation steps. In general, the binding between these layers involves different types of chemical interactions of the functional (head-) groups of the distinct interfaces. One reason for multilayers is that only an even number of LB-films coated onto an ultraflat hydrophilic surface (mica, silica) is stable under water. LB-films often offer the best film in terms of flatness and total amount of surface coating. However, since these layers are only relatively weak bound onto the supporting surface the first layer can be coated, for example, by a covalently bound silane and the second layer by LB-technique.

The two major interactions employed for immobilizing biological specimens to solid supports are physisorption, i.e. an immobilization entirely due to non-covalent interactions, and chemisorption, i.e. immobilization through covalent chemical bonds. Most of the results discussed in the context of this thesis are based on coating the supporting surface by self-assembled monolayers. Most popular are alkanthiols which grow spontaneously on epitactic (hydrophilic) Au(111) films, or silanes (aminosilylated silica) that are deposited from the liquid or gas phase onto silica. Amphiphiles transferred onto a solid support by employing the LB-technique might offer the highest quality of deposited films in terms of flatness and chemical purity of the coating film or layers. When starting with a hydrophilic surface an even number of transferred monolayers is required for the stability of the outermost lipid layer under liquid. However, for some amphiphiles the deposition of a second monolayer with an overall low defect rate can be quite difficult to achieve. During the downstroke through the air-water interface when using the LB-technique a variety of different forces are acting on the interface region between subphase, air and supporting substrate. In fact sometimes the initial layer is readily stripped off because of it being non-covalently bound to the substrate. In contrast, by employing the monolayer method the hydrophobic surface of the highly oriented pyrolytic graphite (HOPG) surface is used to directly transfer the alkane chains with the arrays of (para-) crystalline proteins grown on the hydrophilic end of the lipids (DNA, actin, porin). A hydrophobic surface is not wetable and a soft sample potentially might be distorted during transfer. However, HOPG is known to potentially produce a wide range of artifacts and therefore might not be the first choice.

2.2.5.4 Examples

2.2.5.4.1 "Spontaneous" adsorption of amyloid-like fibrils

Prior to imaging the sample needs to stably adsorb to a solid support and hence it has to come in close contact with the support surface. A number of water soluble peptides that form fibrils similar to those comprising amyloid deposits of Alzheimer's and Creuzfeld-Jacob disease patients get trapped on mica but also on HOPG and by LB-film modified mica surface comprising positive, neutral and negative charges (unpublished data). Most work was done on mica surfaces were the nucleation, elongation, branching and lateral association of individual amyloid-like fibrils were followed by time-lapse AFM over several hours in physiological buffer environment. Fibril growth may be recorded in TM AFM or in CM AFM (Goldsbury et al. 1999; Stolz et al. 2000).

2.2.5.4.2 Adsorption of 2D membranes by electrostatic balancing

Biological membranes constituting of 2D crystalline arrays of a membrane protein patched into a lipid bilayer are ideal specimens for being imaged by AFM, as they are relatively "smooth", i.e. their surface corrugation are in the nanometer range. Because of their 2D crystalline nature optimizing the parameters for operating the AFM is relatively easy. For their immobilization different methods were employed and developed, i.e. in one protocol the sample was cross-linked to a functionalized glass surface, i.e. coverslips were chemically modified with the photoactive cross-linker N-5-azido-2-nitrobenzoyloxysuccinimide (Karrasch et al. 1994). Another strategy supports the adsorption of the membrane patches while overcoming the repulsive forces by saturating the surface charges so that the attractive forces between support and specimen become predominant (Shao et al. 2000). Often a net attractive force to adsorb those membranes can thus be achieved by adjusting the pH and the salt concentration of mono- or divalent salts within the buffer until the appropriate amount of counterions are present in the buffer to optimize the adsorption behavior (Muller et al. 1999a; Wagner 1998). To achieve this, membrane patches suspended in buffer are applied to freshly cleaved mica by injecting them into a buffer droplet. After adsorption for typically 10-15 minutes most of the membrane patches or some other supramolecular assemblies are strongly adhering to the mica surface.

2.2.5.4.3 Adsorption of actin arrays by adjusting the appropriate surface charge

Sometimes the immobilization strategy by electrostatic balancing for adsorbing biolomolecules is not applicable, because of the instability of the sample. G- and F-actin polymers and 2D crystalline arrays discussed later in this thesis are formed in buffers that require very stringent pH, ionic strength and multivalent cation conditions, so that relatively small alterations in the ion content may cause disassembly of these specimens. Hence, it is important to find the "optimal" support surface conditions that yield stable adsorption and yet do not cause disassembly of the distinct actin crystalline arrays. The most important prerequisites are the appropriate strength of charge together with a sufficiently flat surface so as to allow for resolution imaging. By producing supported LB-films on a freshly cleaved mica surface by an appropriate mixture of cationic lipids of cationic (i.e. DDDMA, Dimethyldioctadecylammonium Bromide) and neutral (i.e. DLPC, 1,2-Dilauroyl-sn-Glycero-3-Phosphocholine) lipids allowed us for the first time to achieve stable adsorption and high resolution imaging of different actin arrays.

2.2.5.4.4 Transfer of 2D protein crystals onto hydrophobic surfaces by the monolayer method

In another strategy 2D protein crystals were directly grown on lipid monolayers that are on top of a droplet of polymerization buffer and then transferred onto a hydrophobic surface support, such as highly oriented pyrolytic graphite (HOPG), for imaging in the AFM. A good example for this so-called monolayer method is streptavidin crystals that were grown on biotinylated lipid monolayers at an air/ water interface before being transferred onto HOPG. Even, stronger hydrophobic surfaces can be produced by the hydrophobic head groups of lipid monolayers transferred onto mica by employing the LB-technique. By using HOPG and mica surfaces modified by a monolayer of arachidic acid ($C_{20}H_{40}O_2$) we successfully immobilized paracrystalline F-actin filament arrays that were grown on a lipid monolayer as described by Taylor and Taylor (Taylor and Taylor 1992). In addition, we employed the HOPG-based monolayer method that has the advantage that it does not require the transfer of a lipid monolayer. We tried preparations that employ the hydrophobic tails of the alkane chains of arachidic acid. Adsorption of F-actin paracrystals to arachidic acid yields a slightly more rigid binding of the sample to the monolayer and consequently to a slightly more stable imaging by the AFM tip. However, the arachidic acid film tends to reorganize into a multilayer when there is not a very dense packing of the paracrystalline F-actin filament arrays is achieved.

2.2.5.4.5 Binding of biomolecules to solid supports by silanization

Plasmid-DNA and protein-DNA complexes are typical most stably to a mica surface after it has been silanized. By this approach the biomolecules can be attached to a functionalized support either directly using various substrates reacted with 3-aminopropyltriethoxysilane (APTES), or indirectly by photochemical cross-linking to immobilized psoralen derivates. Covalent attachment of biomolecules to the solid support surface also allows reproducible imaging of DNA. Binding of biomolecules to solid supports by silanization works for many biomolecules, but in particular for DNA so that reproducible high-resolution imaging is achieved.

2.2.5.4.6 Stable adsorption of Xenopus oocyte envelopes

Our goal here was to reproducibly and at the highest possible resolution imaging of NPCs by AFM. The pores in the cell nucleus, the nuclear pore complexes (NPC) residing in the double-membrane nuclear envelope (NE) were investigated. The nucleus of the Xenopus oocyte is of macroscopically dimensions, i.e. it has a diameter of 0.3 – 0.5 mm. The diameter of a single pore imbedded in the membrane is about 120 nm, the height at the cytoplasmic side is about 35 nm above the membrane surface, whereas the height of the basket at the nuclear side is about 70 nm. Therefore the overall height of the whole specimen is roughly about 100 nm. Hence the requirement for the specimen support in terms of its corrugation is not as stringent as it has to be for imaging crystalline arrays of membrane proteins or actin filament arrays at high resolution. For AFM imaging Xenopus oocyte NEs that had not been exposed to any detergents or chemical fixatives were spread on EM that were coated with a glow-discharged carbon film (Aebi and Pollard 1987). This way either the cytoplasmic or the nuclear surface of spread NEs could be prepared for AFM imaging at a resolution of 20-30 nm. Although the thus prepared NEs were very soft no gain in resolution was achieved by TM AFM over CM AFM.

2.2.5.4.6 Preparing articular cartilage for AFM imaging

For AFM imaging of cartilage with sharp pyramidal tips pieces of cartilage, about ~5 mm x 5 mm x 2 mm in size, were cut with a sharp razor blade from the medial and lateral condyles of the femoral side of the knee joint.

For imaging under buffer solution, the outermost ~1 mm thick cartilage layer parallel to the support surface of the cartilage surface were discarded with a vibratory microtome (752 M Vibroslice, Campden Instruments, Loughborough, UK) to image the middle section of full thickness blocks.

For imaging in air the tissue blocks of articular porcine cartilage were imbedded and sectioned with a cryostat (SLEE, Mainz, Germany) at -15 °C. The outermost 300 - 500 μm of the cartilage surface were discarded to minimize surface irregularities and to harvest the cartilage from middle section of full thickness blocks. 20 μm thick frozen sections were then adsorbed to glass cover slips (6 mm diameter) that had been coated with a 0.01% Poly-L-Lysine solution (Sigma, P8920) solution dried in an oven at 60°C. After adsorption, the sections were dried on a hotplate at 40°C. Images were recorded under buffer solution or in air in contact mode AFM. Imaging under buffer solution hardly resolved individual fibers of the collagen network, whereas imaging in air clearly resolved their 67 nm axial repeat distance of individual fibrils.

2.2.5.4.7 Preparation articular cartilage for elasticity measurements

For elasticity measurements cartilage samples were prepared from porcine tibial heads by cutting out small blocks of ~5 mm x 5 mm x 2 mm. These cartilage blocks were mounted on a stainless steel supported Teflon® disc with Histoacryl® tissue glue (B. Braun Surgical GmbH, 34209 Melsungen, Germany). To obtain a smooth and flat specimen surface the mounted cartilage blocks were slightly trimmed parallel to the support surface in a vibratory microtome.

By employing indentation-type AFM (IT AFM) biomechanical parameters can be conducted. In this operational mode the tip was placed directly atop individual structural features and the deflection of the cantilever was recorded by an optical detection system during one whole loading-unloading cycle, i.e. while the sample was pushed against and retracted from the tip. Some important biomechanical properties of the sample such as hardness, elasticity, viscoelasticity, plasticity could thus be reflected in the load-indentation curves and at high precision, i.e. the optical detection system allowed recording of 0.1 nm displacement resolution (in Z-direction) corresponding to forces up to 10 pN (Shao et al. 1996). These load-indentation curves then eventually allowed conducting the biomechanical parameter of interest by means of a model or by providing a reference measurement on a standard with a known mechanical property.

Later on in this thesis I demonstrate that the determination of the elastic modulus of biological matter at two different scales, i.e. by employing nanometer sized tips or by employing micrometer sized tips, eventually leads to fundamentally different elastic moduli as recorded on biological tissues. For example, the elastic modulus obtained at porcine articular cartilage when measured at the (sub-) cellular scale (nanometer sized tips) resulted in a 100-fold lower elastic modulus as measured at the overall tissue level (micrometer sized tips) and at the same sample.

It is proposed that those two fundamentally different elasticity values reflect the multi-component and multi-phasic nature of this highly complex cartilage tissue. This hypothesis was supported by a series of digestion experiments that systematically degraded distinct components of the extracellular matrix, such as proteoglycans, glycoaminoglycans or the collagen fibrils, of the cartilage architecture in a specific manner thereby altering the elastical properties of the tissue in a very specific manner.

2.2.5.5 Imaging biological specimens by AFM

The prerequisite for membrane proteins to be imaged at high resolution by AFM is that they occur as densely packed, well-ordered two-dimensional (2D) crystalline arrays *in vivo*, or else have been reconstituted into phospholipid bilayers to form highly ordered 2D crystalline arrays *in vitro*. The adhesion of there 2D crystalline arrays to the support and 2D crystalline packing of the membrane proteins within a lipid bilayer provide the lateral stability that is necessary for scanning the specimen with the AFM tip. Therefore the individual proteins do not necessarily require a strong affinity for the support, as it is the contact area of the entire 2D crystalline array that eventually yield stable immobilization of the specimen to the support. Highest resolution can only be achieved by minimizing long-range forces acting between the tip and the sample surface, i.e. by adjusting the pH ionic strength of the surrounding buffer. More specifically, the choice of the electrolyte determines the electrostatic interaction between the negatively charged pyramidal Si_3N_4 tip and the sample surface. To achieve optimal resolution the ionic strength has to be such that the tip slides over the protein surface by exerting a minimal lateral force onto the sample.

By employing this method most remarkable resolution so far is achieved by employing membrane proteins arrays such as hexagonally packed intermediate (HPI) layer from Deinoccocus radiodurans (Karrasch et al. 1994), cholera toxin (Mou et al. 1995), OmpF porin from Escheria coli (Muller et al. 1997), and the bacteriorhodopsin from Halobacterium salinarium (Muller et al. 1999b). A resolution of 10 Å, 1 to 2 nm, 8 Å and ~5 Å, respectively have been achieved.

The ionic strength for achieving stable adsorption of the specimen to the support may be different from the optimal electrolyte needed for obtaining highest-resolution imaging. For example, depending on whether the asymmetric unit membrane (AUM) of the bladder urothelium shall preferentially adsorbed with its luminal or cytoplasmic face, different ionic strength are required. By optimizing the respective adsorption conditions to mica supports, both the luminal and cytoplasmic surface of the 16-nm AUM plaque particles could be imaged with spatial resolution of 15 Å.

2.3 References

Aebi U, Pollard TD. 1987. A glow discharge unit to render electron microscope grids and other surfaces hydrophilic. *J Electron Microsc Tech* 7(1):29-33.

Amos LA, Huxley HE, Holmes KC, Goody RS, Taylor KA. 1982. Structural evidence that myosin heads may interact with two sites on f-actin. *Nature* 299(5882):467-9.

Appleyard RC, Swain MV, Khanna S, Murrell GA. 2001. The accuracy and reliability of a novel handheld dynamic indentation probe for analysing articular cartilage. *Phys Med Biol* 46(2):541-50.

Aspden RM, Larsson T, Svensson R, Heinegard D. 1991. Computer-controlled mechanical testing machine for small samples of biological viscoelastic materials. *J Biomed Eng* 13(6):521-5.

Bader DL, Kempson GE. 1994. The short-term compressive properties of adult human articular cartilage. *Biomed Mater Eng* 4(3):245-56.

Bader DL, Kempson GE, Egan J, Gilbey W, Barrett AJ. 1992. The effects of selective matrix degradation on the short-term compressive properties of adult human articular cartilage. *Biochim Biophys Acta* 1116(2):147-54.

Binnig G, Quate CF, Gerber C. 1986. Atomic force microscope. *Physical Review Letters* vol.56, no.9; 3 March 1986; p.930 3.

Binnig G, Rohrer H. 1982. Scanning tunnelling microscopy. *Helvetica Physica Acta* vol.55, no.6; 1982; p.726 35.

Chothia C, Lesk AM. 1986. The relation between the divergence of sequence and structure in proteins. *Embo J* 5(4):823-6.

Chothia C, Lesk AM, Levitt M, Amit AG, Mariuzza RA, Phillips SE, Poljak RJ. 1986. The predicted structure of immunoglobulin d1.3 and its comparison with the crystal structure. *Science* 233(4765):755-8.

Cohen NP, Foster RJ, Mow VC. 1998. Composition and dynamics of articular cartilage: Structure, function, and maintaining healthy state. *J Orthop Sports Phys Ther* 28(4):203-15.

DiBella LM, King SM. 2001. Dynein motors of the chlamydomonas flagellum. *Int Rev Cytol* 210:227-68.

Engel A, Gaub HE, Muller DJ. 1999. Atomic force microscopy: A forceful way with single molecules. *Curr Biol* 9(4):R133-6.

Ernst RR, Bodenhausen G, Wolkaun A. 1987. Principles of nuclear magnetic resonance in one and two dimensions. *Clarendon Press* Oxford.

Franz T, Hasler EM, Hagg R, Weiler C, Jakob RP, Mainil-Varlet P. 2001. In situ compressive stiffness, biochemical composition, and structural integrity of articular cartilage of the human knee joint. *Osteoarthritis Cartilage* 9(6):582-92.

Goldsbury C, Kistler J, Aebi U, Arvinte T, Cooper GJ. 1999. Watching amyloid fibrils grow by time-lapse atomic force microscopy. *J Mol Biol* 285(1):33-9.

Grimm R, Singh H, Rachel R, Typke D, Zillig W, Baumeister W. 1998. Electron tomography of ice-embedded prokaryotic cells. *Biophys J* 74(2 Pt 1):1031-42

Guss JM, Merritt EA, Phizackerley RP, Hedman B, Murata M, Hodgson KO, Freeman HC. 1988. Phase determination by multiple-wavelength X-ray diffraction: Crystal structure of a basic "blue" copper protein from cucumbers. *Science* 241(4867):806-11.

Hansma HG, Laney DE, Bezanilla M, Sinsheimer RL, Hansma PK. 1995. Applications for atomic force microscopy of DNA. *Biophys J* 68(5):1672-7.

Hayes WC, Keer LM, Herrmann G, Mockros LF. 1972. A mathematical analysis for indentation tests of articular cartilage. *J Biomech* 5(5):541-51.

Hegner M, Wagner P, Semenza G. 1993. Immobilizing DNA on gold via thiol modification for atomic force microscopy imaging in buffer solutions. *FEBS Lett* 336(3): 452-6.

Henderson R, Unwin PN. 1975. Three-dimensional model of purple membrane obtained by electron microscopy. *Nature* 257(5521):28-32.

Hendrickson WA. 1991. Determination of macromolecular structures from anomalous diffraction of synchrotron radiation. *Science* 254(5028):51-8.

Hoenger A, Sablin EP, Vale RD, Fletterick RJ, Milligan RA. 1995. Three-dimensional structure of a tubulin-motor-protein complex. *Nature* 376(6537):271-4.

Jurvelin JS, Arokoski JP, Hunziker EB, Helminen HJ. 2000. Topographical variation of the elastic properties of articular cartilage in the canine knee. *J Biomech* 33(6):669-75.

Kaab MJ, Ito K, Clark JM, Notzli HP. 2000. The acute structural changes of loaded articular cartilage following meniscectomy or acl-transection. *Osteoarthritis Cartilage* 8(6):464-73.

Kachar B, Liang F, Lins U, Ding M, Wu XR, Stoffler D, Aebi U, Sun TT. 1999. Three-dimensional analysis of the 16 nm urothelial plaque particle: Luminal surface exposure, preferential head-to-head interaction, and hinge formation. *J Mol Biol* 285(2): 595-608.

Karrasch S, Hegerl R, Hoh JH, Baumeister W, Engel A. 1994. Atomic force microscopy produces faithful high-resolution images of protein surfaces in an aqueous environment. *Proc Natl Acad Sci U S A* 91(3):836-8.

Langer R, Vacanti JP. 1993. Tissue engineering. *Science* 260(5110):920-6.

Mancini EJ, de Haas F, Fuller SD. 1997. High-resolution icosahedral reconstruction: Fulfilling the promise of cryo-electron microscopy. *Structure* 5(6):741-50.

McDevitt CA, Muir H. 1976. Biochemical changes in the cartilage of the knee in experimental and natural osteoarthritis in the dog. *J Bone Joint Surg Br* 58(1):94-101.

Miles M. 1997. Scanning probe microscopy. Probing the future. *Science* 277(5333):1845-7.

Min G, Stolz M, Zhou G, Liang F, Sebbel P, Stoffler D, Glockshuber R, Sun TT, Aebi U, Kong XP. 2002. Localization of uroplakin ia, the urothelial receptor for bacterial adhesion fimh, on the six inner domains of the 16 nm urothelial plaque particle. *J. Mol. Biol* 317(5):697-706.

Miyatani T, Horii M, Rosa A, Fujihira M. 1997. Mapping of electrical double-layer force between tip and sample surfaces in water with pulsed-force-mode atomic force microscopy. *Applied Physics Letters* vol.71, no.18; p.2632 4.

Mogilner A, Fisher AJ, Baskir RJ. 2001. Structural changes in the neck linker of kinesin explain the load dependence of the motor's mechanical cycle. *J Theor Biol* 211(2): 143-57.

Moller C, Allen M, Elings V, Engel A, Muller DJ. 1999. Tapping-mode atomic force microscopy produces faithful high-resolution images of protein surfaces. *Biophys J* 77(2):1150-8.

Mou J, Yang J, Shao Z. 1995. Atomic force microscopy of cholera toxin b-oligomers bound to bilayers of biologically relevant lipids. *J Mol Biol* 248(3):507-12.

Muller DJ, Fotiadis D, Scheuring S, Muller SA, Engel A. 1999a. Electrostatically balanced subnanometer imaging of biological specimens by atomic force microscope. *Biophys J* 76(2):1101-11.

Muller DJ, Sass HJ, Muller SA, Buldt G, Engel A. 1999b. Surface structures of native bacteriorhodopsin depend on the molecular packing arrangement in the membrane. *J Mol Biol* 285(5):1903-9.

Muller DJ, Schoenenberger CA, Schabert F, Engel A. 1997. Structural changes in native membrane proteins monitored at subnanometer resolution with the atomic force microscope: A review. *Journal of Structural Biology* 119:149-157.

Opalka N, Tihova M, Brugidou C, Kumar A, Beachy RN, Fauquet CM, Yeager M. 2000. Structure of native and expanded sobemoviruses by electron cryo-microscopy and image reconstruction. *J Mol Biol* 303(2):197-211.

Peppas NA, Langer R. 1994. New challenges in biomaterials. *Science* 263(5154):1715-20.

Putman CA, van der Werf KO, de Grooth BG, van Hulst NF, Greve J. 1994. Viscoelasticity of living cells allows high resolution imaging by tapping mode atomic force microscopy. *Biophys J* 67(4):1749-53.

Richardson JW, Jacobson RA. 1987. "patterson and pattersons" (j. P. Glusker, b. K. Patterson, and m. Rossi, eds.), p. 310. I.U.Cr. And o.U.P., oxford.

Roth V, Mow VC. 1980. The intrinsic tensile behavior of the matrix of bovine articular cartilage and its variation with age. *J Bone Joint Surg Am* 62(7):1102-17.

Rubenstein JD, Li JG, Majumdar S, Henkelman RM. 1997. Image resolution and signal-to-noise ratio requirements for mr imaging of degenerative cartilage. *AJR Am J Roentgenol* 169(4):1089-96.

Ruiz T, Erk I, Lepault J. 1994. Electron cryo-microscopy of vitrified biological specimens: Towards high spatial and temporal resolution. *Biol Cell* 80(2-3):203-10.

Salisbury SA, Wilson SE, Powell HR, Kennard O, Lubini P, Sheldrick GM, Escaja N, Alazzouzi E, Grandas A, Pedroso E. 1997. The bi-loop, a new general four-stranded DNA motif. *Proc Natl Acad Sci U S A* 94(11):5515-8.

Schoenenberger CA, Hoh JH. 1994. Slow cellular dynamics in mdck and r5 cells monitored by time-lapse atomic force microscopy. *Biophys J* 67(2):929-36.

Schoenenberger CA, Steinmetz MO, Stoffler D, Mandinova A, Aebi U. 1999. Structure, assembly, and dynamics of actin filaments in situ and in vitro. *Microsc Res Tech* 47(1):38-50.

Schroder RR, Manstein DJ, Jahn W, Holden H, Rayment I, Holmes KC, Spudich JA. 1993. Three-dimensional atomic model of f-actin decorated with dictyostelium myosin s1. *Nature* 364(6433):171-4.

Shao Z, Mou J, Czajkowsky DM, Yang J, Yuan J-Y. 1996. Biological atomic force microscopy: What is achieved and what is needed. *Advances in Physics* vol.45, no.1; Jan. Feb. 1996; p.1 86.

Shao Z, Shi D, Somlyo AV. 2000. Cryoatomic force microscopy of filamentous actin. *Biophys J* 78(2):950-8.

Sheldrick GM, Jones PG, Kennard O, Williams DH, Smith GA. 1978. Structure of vancomycin and its complex with acetyl-d-alanyl-d-alanine. *Nature* 271(5642):223-5.

Shepherd DE, Seedhom BB. 1997. A technique for measuring the compressive modulus of articular cartilage under physiological loading rates with preliminary results. *Proc Inst Mech Eng [H]* 211(2):155-65.

Shih WM, Gryczynski Z, Lakowicz JR, Spudich JA. 2000. A fret-based sensor reveals large atp hydrolysis-induced conformational changes and three distinct states of the molecular motor myosin. *Cell* 102(5):683-94.

Sinclair DA, Smith IR, Wickramasinghe HK, McAvoy BR. 1982. Elastic constants measurement in the acoustic microscope. *Ultrasonics Symposium Proceedings* IEEE, New York, NY, USA; 1982; 2 vol. 1090 pp.

Stoffler D, Steinmetz MO, Aebi U. 1999. Imaging biological matter across dimensions: From cells to molecules and atoms. *Faseb J* 13 Suppl 2:S195-200.

Stolz M, Seidel J, Martin I, Raiteri R, Aebi U, Baschong W. 1999. Ex vivo measurement of the elasticity of extracellular matrix constituents by atomic force microscopy (afm). *Mol. Biol. Cell 10, 145a.*

Stolz M, Stoffler D, Aebi U, Goldsbury C. 2000. Monitoring biomolecular interactions by time-lapse atomic force microscopy. *J Struct Biol* 131(3):171-80.

Taylor KA, Taylor DW. 1992. Formation of 2-d paracrystals of f-actin on phospholipid layers mixed with quaternary ammonium surfactants. *J Struct Biol* 108(2):140-7.

Tkaczuk H. 1986. Human cartilage stiffness. In vivo studies. *Clin Orthop*(206):301-12.

Unwin PN, Henderson R. 1975. Molecular structure determination by electron microscopy of unstained crystalline specimens. *J Mol Biol* 94(3):425-40.

Vale RD, Milligan RA. 2000. The way things move: Looking under the hood of molecular motor proteins. *Science* 288(5463):88-95.

Voges D, Berendes R, Burger A, Demange P, Baumeister W, Huber R. 1994. Three-dimensional structure of membrane-bound annexin v. A correlative electron microscopy-X-ray crystallography study. *J Mol Biol* 238(2):199-213.

Vunjak-Novakovic G, Martin I, Obradovic B, Treppo S, Grodzinsky AJ, Langer R, Freed LE. 1999. Bioreactor cultivation conditions modulate the composition and mechanical properties of tissue-engineered cartilage. *J Orthop Res* 17(1):130-8.

Wagner P. 1998. Immobilization strategies for biological scanning probe microscopy. *FEBS Lett* 430(1-2):112-5.

Wagner P, Hegner M, Kernen P, Zaugg F, Semenza G. 1996. Covalent immobilization of native biomolecules onto au(111) via n-hydroxysuccinimide ester functionalized self-assembled monolayers for scanning probe microscopy. *Biophys J* 70(5):2052-66.

Wagner P, Kernen P, Hegner M, Ungewickell E, Semenza G. 1994. Covalent anchoring of proteins onto gold-directed nhs-terminated self-assembled monolayers in aqueous buffers: Sfm images of clathrin cages and triskelia. *FEBS Lett* 356(2-3):267-71.

Walz T, Haner M, Wu XR, Henn C, Engel A, Sun TT, Aebi U. 1995. Towards the molecular architecture of the asymmetric unit membrane of the mammalian urinary bladder epithelium: A closed "twisted ribbon" structure. *J Mol Biol* 248(5): 887-900.

Wu XR, Sun TT, Medina JJ. 1996. In vitro binding of type 1-fimbriated escherichia coli to uroplakins ia and ib: Relation to urinary tract infections. *Proc Natl Acad Sci U S A* 93(18):9630-5.

3. Asymmetric Unit Membrane

3 Imaging the luminal and cytoplasmic face of the asymmetric unit membrane (AUM) by atomic force microscopy (AFM) in their functional state

The mammalian bladder is a highly complex and vital system, which naturally undergoes large conformational changes. The AUM serves as the surface of the bladder and functions as a physical barrier to urine. Additionally, the AUM is one of the few examples of a biological membrane that forms 2D crystals *in situ*. Hence, the AUM is an excellent model system for investigating structural changes (1) at the level of formation and rearrangement of AUM plaques, and (2) at the level of single plaque particles. As a prerequisite for tracking the formation of plaques by time-lapse AFM and to eventually investigate different conformations of individual particles, we developed a protocol for the stable immobilization of AUM plaques onto a mica surface in their native state. As a result, we succeeded to image both the luminal and cytoplasmic faces of the AUM with a resolution of ~1.5 nm. Moreover, the AUM exhibited a clear crystalline arrangement at both faces. In addition, the AFM permitted to accurately measure the heights of both surfaces, absolute and relative to the embedding lipid bilayer. Finally, we compared our AFM surface topographies gathered under native buffer conditions with novel 3D reconstructions computed both from negatively stained and ice-embedded AUM plaques (Min et al. 2002; Oostergetel et al. 2001).

3.1 Introduction

The bladder epithelium is almost entirely covered with numerous plaques characterized by a luminal leaflet being much thicker than the cytoplasmic one, hence the name "asymmetric unit membrane" or AUM. The AUM consists of distinct, rigid looking plaque, typically 0.2 µm to 1 µm in diameters, which are interspersed by so-called "hinge" regions. Each individual AUM plaque is a 2D hexagonal crystal (i.e. exhibiting P_6 two-sided plane group symmetry) made of distinct, 16 nm spaced particles. These so-called 16-nm plaque particles are embedded in a lipid bilayer membrane. Despite the fact that the AUM has been investigated structurally for over 30 years, the cytoplasmic surface has so far resisted imaging so as to directly exhibit the hexagonal packing of the plaque particles.

However, unidirectionally shadowed replicas of unfixed, quick-frozen/ freeze-fractured AUMs indicated a periodic structure being present on their cytoplasmic face (Kachar et al. 1999). As yet, little is known about the functional aspects of the AUM, neither at the level of individual plaques nor at the level of single plaque particles (Kachar et al. 1999).

It has been speculated that a function of the plaque particles might be stabilization of the luminal surface. Moreover, it was suggested that they might contribute to the remarkable permeability barrier function of the urothelium, to the reversible adjustment of the apical surface area, and to the physical stabilization of the apical surface during bladder distention (Lewis 2000; Sun et al. 1999).

Morphological analysis of urothelial plaques has indicated that they are dynamic structures that in response to mechanical strains and stress change their size and shape by the disappearance of existing and reappearance of new hinges separating adjacent plaques (Kachar et al. 1999). In the context of tracking the dynamic behavior of these AUM plaques the AFM is the instrument of choice with the capability to directly image the surface topography of biological samples that are kept in a near-physiological buffer environment at sub-nm resolution (Muller et al. 1995; Schabert et al. 1995). Moreover, the AFM allows to measure the surface elevations and depressions of biological samples with a precision of a few tens of nanometers (Engel et al. 1999; Shao et al. 1996). Hence, we employed the AFM for determining the luminal surface topography of the plaque particles and also for trying to directly visualize the putative cytoplasmic protrusions of the transmembrane helices anchoring the plaque particles in the bladder membrane.

3.2 Materials and Methods

3.2.1 Materials

Unless specified otherwise, all chemicals were of analytical or best available grade and purchased from Sigma Chemie AG (Buchs, Switzerland). For all experiments and buffers, ultrapure deionized water was used (18 MΩ/cm; Brandstead, Boston, USA). The buffers used were either Tris or Hepes with the pH of all buffers being adjusted at room temperature.

3.2.2 Isolation and negative staining of AUM plaques

Bovine and mouse urothelial AUM plaques were isolated by sucrose density gradient centrifugation and differential detergent washing (Liang et al. 1999; Wu et al. 1990). For negative staining, 5 ml of an AUM sample (typically 0.1 mg/ml in storage buffer consisting of 15 mM Hepes-NaOH, pH 7.5, 1 mM EDTA and 1mM EGTA) was applied to a freshly glow-discharged carbon film (Aebi and Pollard 1987) supported by a copper grid (300 meshes), and the adsorbed AUM plaques were then negatively stained using 0.75% uranyl formate, pH 4.25. In some experiments, the storage buffer contained in addition 0.02% to 0.2% Triton X-100.

3.2.3 Image recording and processing

Negatively stained AUM samples were examined using a Philips CM200 FEG transmission electron microscope operated at 200 kV. Micrographs of AUM plaques that were > 0.5 µm in diameter were taken in a low dose mode at 50,000X. After the low dose image was taken, each plaque was examined using a CCD camera, excluding those plaques that were folded or double-layered. For 3D reconstruction, tilted images were recorded at 0, 20, 30, 45 and 55 degrees. Since the crystals have P_6 symmetry, samples were tilted only in one direction. The micrographs were screened using an optical diffractometer to select the regions that yielded the highest resolution diffraction spots (better than 20 Å). The selected micrographs were then scanned using a PDS microdensitometer using a step size of 20 µm, which corresponds to 4 Å in the crystal. After the digitized images were transferred to SGI computers, they were corrected for long-range disorder, merged and used to calculate the averaged projection maps using the MRC software suites (Crowther et al. 1996; Henderson et al. 1990) and CCP4 (CCP4 1994). After correction of any lattice distortions, the images were trimmed to 2600 x 2600 pixels so that they contained > 1000 unit cells. The final 3D density was displayed using the program "O".

3.2.4 Atomic force microscopy

All AFM measurements were performed with a Nanoscope III (Digital Instruments, Santa Barbara, CA) equipped with a 120-µm scanner (J-scanner) and a fluid cell. Oxide sharpened silicon nitride cantilevers with a nominal spring constant of 0.06 N/m from Digital Instruments were used. Before use, the fluid cell was cleaned with normal dish cleaner, followed by ethanol and finally ultrapure water rinsing. Small disks, ~5 mm in diameter, were punched out of mica (Mica New York Corp., New York) and glued with water insoluble epoxy glue (Araldit, Ciba Geigy AG, Basel, Switzerland) onto a Teflon disc that, in turn, was supported by a slightly smaller diameter steel disc. The steel disc is required so that the specimen can be mounted magnetically onto the piezoelectric scanner. Sample preparation

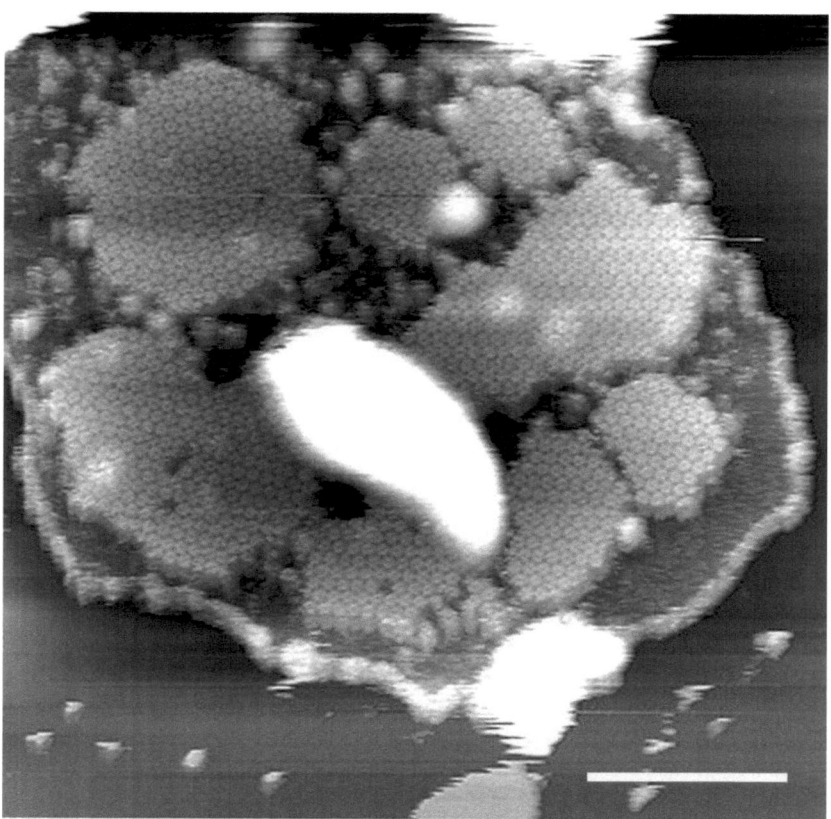

FIGURE 1: Measurement of the absolute heights of the AUM. All height measurements were provided on stable immobilized urothelial plaques at a mica surface in a close to native buffer environment. The overall height of the entire urothelial plaque was measured to ~12.5 nm; the height of the lipid membrane is ~5.5 nm; the leaflet above the lipid bilayer at the luminal side raised by ~6.5 nm above the luminal membrane surface and the donut-shaped protrusions of the cytoplasmic side is ~0.5 nm above the lipid membrane. Scale bar, 250 nm.

for AFM was done by placing 2-μl aliquots of AUM onto a freshly cleaved piece of mica. To achieve stable adsorption for imaging the luminal membrane surface, storage buffer (10 mM Hepes-NaOH pH 7.5) was used. In contrast, when aiming to image the cytoplasmic membrane surface, i.e. to stably adsorb the AUM plaques with their luminal face to the mica surface, we used 10 mM Tris-HCl, pH 8.5, 250 mM KCl. After about 15 minutes of adsorption the sample was gently washed with the buffer used for imaging to remove non-adsorbed membranes. Both surfaces were imaged in the same buffer; i.e. 10 mM Hepes, pH 7.5, 250 mM KCl. All AFM imaging was performed in contact mode and at a scan speed of ~5.5 Hz.

3.3 Results and Discussion

3.3.1 Height measurements of the AUM

The AFM allowed us to measure the heights of the crystalline leaflets protruding from either side of the lipid bilayer with a precision that was limited by the corrugation of the soft biological surface which is about 2 Å (Fig. 1). Accordingly, the AUM exhibited an overall height of ~12.5 nm (i.e. measured from the mica support), i.e. the thickness of the lipid membrane of ~5.5 nm, the height of the luminal leaflet protruding by ~6.5 nm above the lipid membrane and the cytoplasmic face that protrudes by ~0.5 nm out of the lipid membrane (see below). These results are in good agreement with data obtained recently by cryo-EM. Those data revealed an overall height of the AUM of ~13.2 nm, the thickness of the lipid bilayer of ~4 nm and the height of the luminal part above the membrane of ~7.2 nm (Oostergetel et al. 2001).

3.3.2 Visualization of fully native urothelial plaques by atomic force microscopy (AFM)

In the context of structural analysis of biological matter the word "native" has been given different meanings regarding EM and AFM. However, maybe the most important goal when preparing and imaging a biological specimen is to retain its native morphology. Biological specimens have a relatively low mass density of about 1.3 g/cm^3 and will barely be depicted in an electron microscope due to the low inherent contrast. For structural detail to be visualized in TEM negative staining is the classical method for contrasting biological material (Unwin 1974). In this method a heavy metal salt with a higher density, i.e. uranyl formate (3.7 g/cm^3) is used to replace the water of the object until, in the dried specimen, all "holes" and "voids" are ideally filled with heavy metal salt, so that the biological specimen moiety is inferred from the resulting "stain exclusion" pattern. In the TEM the heavy metal stain therefore causes increased elastic scattering of the electrons which, in turn, delineates the "replica" with high contrast.

Fig. 2 compares images as obtained by TEM and AFM of AUM plaque particles of the luminal side exhibited at the same magnification. In contrast to the TEM micrograph the AFM image exhibits more structural detail as a consequence of the higher signal-to-noise (S/N) ratio provided by the AFM. Therefore the AFM offers the direct monitoring of single particle events, i.e. without further image processing to enhance the S/N ratio. Hence, biological relevant static and dynamical processes, such as conformational changes might be directly

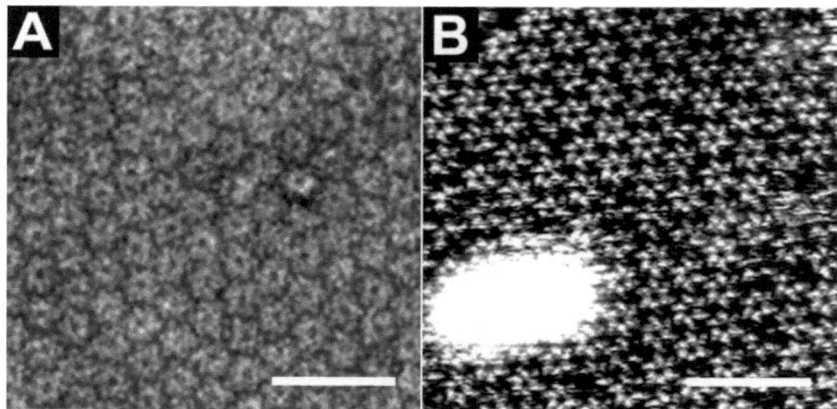

FIGURE 2: Comparison of unprocessed images from urothelial plaque particles as obtained by TEM and AFM (A) Electron micrograph of urothelial plaque particles that were negatively stained with 0.75% uranyl formate. (B) Image of these 16 nm AUM plaque particles that could be readily visualized by AFM with high fidelity even without averaging under native buffer solution. Because of the higher signal-to-noise ratio the AFM image exhibits more structural detail as obtained by TEM. Scale bar, 100 nm.

visualized at the level of single plaque particles as this has previously been demonstrated by the calcium-mediated opening and closing of nuclear pore complexes (NPCs) (Stoffler et al. 1999). Similar to the opening and closing of individual NPCs conformational changes of single plaque particles of the AUM might be induced by physical or chemical effectors and stimuli and therefore depicted by means of time-lapse AFM.

Due to the dehydration of the specimen and the precipitation/ aggregation of inherently soluble components, negative staining harbors a variety of potential artifacts. For example, larger, i.e. sheet-, rod- or tube-like specimens often appear different in the TEM compared to their native state due to effects of spread flattening and/ or collapse during specimen preparation (Bremer et al. 1992; Hoenger and Aebi 1996). But also smaller structures such as negatively stained actin filaments can vary considerably both with respect to morphology and width.

Cryo-EM and the more recently developed cryo-EM tomography are often described as powerful methods for studying the structure, assembly and dynamics of macromolecules and their interactions with substrates in a native-like environment. Indeed, compared to negatively stained samples cryo-EM is able to preserve the biological matter in a much closer to native state (Hoenger and Aebi 1996). Despite these obvious advantages, cryo-EM can only provide "snap shots" of biological specimens that are frozen and therefore immobilized in a layer of vitrified ice. Consequently, the "native state" is already closer to the living state.

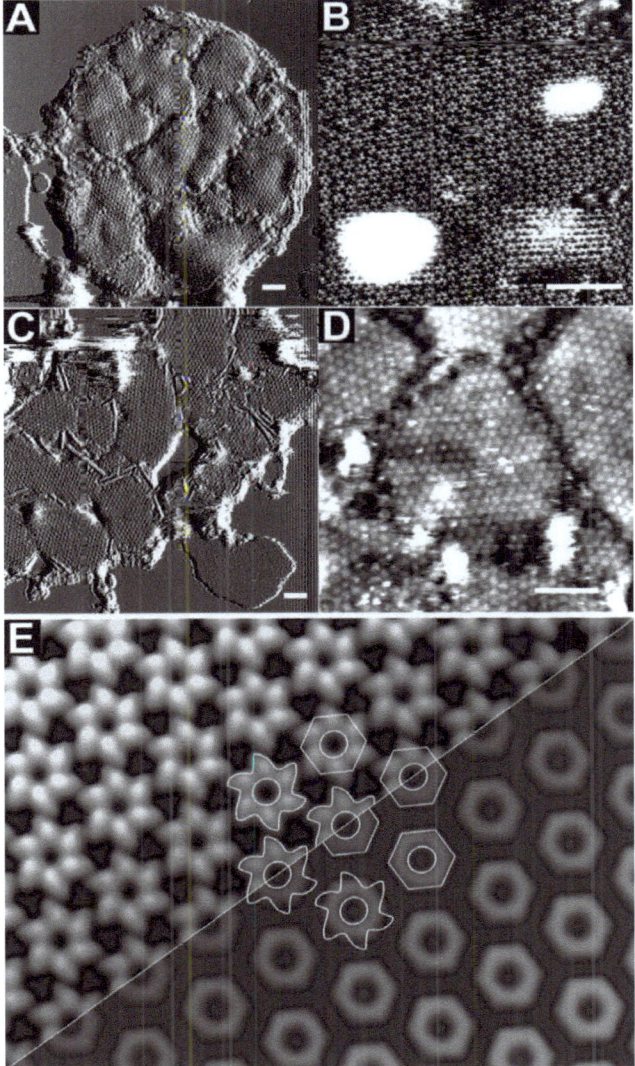

FIGURE 3: Visualization of urothelial plaques by atomic force microscopy. (A) Low magnification view of the luminal face of several bovine urothelial plaques. (B) High magnification view of the luminal surface of a bovine urothelial plaque. Note the hexagonally packed 16 nm AUM particles that could be readily visualized even without averaging. (C) Low magnification view of the cytoplasmic face of several bovine urothelial plaques. Rod-like structures are visible that might be involved of the anchoring of the AUM to the underlying keratin network. (D) High magnification view of the cytoplasmic face of several bovine urothelial plaques. Note the presence of rather flat, donut-like protrusions. (E) The averaged images of the luminal (upper left half in red) and cytoplasmic (lower right half in blue) surfaces of bovine and mouse, respectively, urothelial plaques. Note the propeller-shaped 16 nm AUM particles on the luminal surface, and the ~14 nm diameter, donut-shaped protrusions on the cytoplasmic surface. Scale bars, 100 nm (A to D).

Probably the most spectacular advances of imaging biological samples have been achieved with the AFM. This success might, at least in part, be based on the development of preparation protocols for AFM that keep the specimen in its native state and hence allow imaging of biological matter in a close-to-native environment at the 1-nm resolution level or even beyond. In addition, when aiming at watching biological matter at work, i.e. to step through distinct functional states of the sample only minimal immobilization of the specimen to its solid support should be attempted so as to minimally interfere with its functionality.

In the present investigation the AFM was used for imaging the luminal and cytoplasmic surfaces of urothelial plaques in a close to native physiological buffer environment. Fig. 3A represents an image of the luminal surface of the AUM as imaged by AFM. This low magnification image depicts scallop-shaped plaques that are interspersed by the hinge regions. These scallop-shaped plaques are characterized by hexagonal arrays of 16 nm particles as demonstrated in Fig. 3A and with higher magnification in Fig. 3B. Similarly, the cytoplasmic surface of the bladder urothelium yielded plaque-shaped arrays of hexagonally patched, rather flat protrusions (Fig. 3, C and D). Moreover, the AFM also resolved the hinge regions on the cytoplasmic side Fig. 3, C and D). The rod-like structures depicted in Fig. 3C might represent keratin filaments that are anchored to the AUM. Most strikingly, AFM images of the cytoplasmic surface revealed, for the first time, arrays of donut-shaped, ~0.5 nm high protrusions that had an outer diameter of ~14 nm (Fig 3, C and D).

Based on this AFM data single particle averaging of both faces of the AUM urothelium was performed by averaging typically 100 particles each. The averaged particles on the luminal surface appear propeller-shaped with an outer diameter of 16 nm Fig. 2E, upper left half (see also Walz, 1995 (Walz et al. 1995)). The overlay of the contour (contour of luminal side onto the cytoplasmic side and vice versa) in Fig. 3E reveals that the cytoplasmic face of the plaque particles appears twisted by roughly 30° relative to its luminal face judged by the relative orientation of the hexagon-like contours of the two particle faces.

3.3.3 Comparison of AFM with negative stain EM and cryo-EM

In contrast to EM, the AFM allows to look at biological matter in its physiological buffer environment, i.e. by keeping the specimen "alive". Moreover, there is a fundamental difference from an information point of view between AFM and EM data: While the AFM data represents a 3D topographical map of the surface, TEM data are 2D through-projections. Hence, the AFM resolves information in z, whereas in the TEM the z information is just "piled up", i.e. unresolved. In contrast, the in-plane (i.e. x, y) resolution obtained by AFM can be worse, ~ the same, or sometimes even better than gathered by TEM, depending on the type of specimen, its mechanical properties, etc.

So far there are two examples were the very high sensitivity and fidelity of recording topographic information of the specimen has been achieved. i.e. to readily detect surface corrugations of a few Å. Examples: (1) the cytoplasmic face of AUM plaques as described in chapters 3.5.2, and (2) the nuclear lamina that adheres to – or is partially being wrapped by the inner nuclear membrane.

More specially: The nuclear lamina, a protein meshwork tightly adhering to the inner nuclear membrane surface, was imaged (i) by EM of freeze-dried/ metal shadowed spread nuclear envelopes (NEs) after treatment with Triton X-100 (Aebi et al. 1986), and (ii) by AFM of fully native (i.e. no chemical fixation, no detergent treatment) spread NEs (Stoffler et al. 1999). AFM images of native NEs revealed a distinct morphology of the meshwork of intermediate-type filaments. The important difference here is the fact that by TEM the lamina meshwork can only be depicted after the nuclear membranes have been "dissolved" by detergent treatment.

From a more general perspective, the AFM allows for obtaining accurate height information of biological specimens, such as biological membranes and as depicted by the height measurements of the distinct parts of the AUM and as demonstrated in chapter 3.5.1.

Another example where AFM was able to obtain more structural detail compared to the EM has been the direct visualization of the "elementary protofilaments" that forms during fibrillation of the hormon peptide amylin into amyloid-like fibrils.

In more detail: Amylin is a peptide hormone that forms fibrillar amyloid deposits in the pancreas of patients that are suffering from late-onset (type 2) diabetes. These amylin containing fibrillar deposits may indeed represent a causative factor in the progression of the disease? By analyzing TEM images of *in vitro* formed amylin fibrils and combining these morphological data with STEM mass measurements of these fibrils, it was postulated that the "elementary protofilament", i.e. the minimal distinct building block of the fibrils, has a diameter of 2-3 nm. While these elementary protofilaments could never be visualized convincingly by TEM, they became readily visible by time-lapse AFM of growing amylin fibrils on a mica support (Goldsbury et al. 2000a; Goldsbury et al. 1997; Goldsbury et al. 2000b).

3.3.4 Structural features of the 16-nm plaque particles as obtained by cryo EM, negative stain EM and AFM

Next, I am comparing structural data on urothelial plaques that have been obtained from 3D reconstructions using cryo-electron crystallography (Oostergetel et al. 2001) with those of 3D reconstruction determined from tilt series of negatively stained (Min et al. 2002). In particular, in their work the two groups, i.e. Oostergetel *et al.* and Min *et al.* focused on the transmembrane moiety and how it protrudes on the cytoplasmic face.

Until now, the cytoplasmic face of urothelial plaques appeared smooth and structureless, by EM of both negatively stained and freeze-dried/ metal-shadowed specimens (Brisson and Wade 1983; Kachar et al. 1999). In contrast, recent freeze fracturing data of the cytoplasmic face indicted some regular but rather small protrusions (Kachar et al. 1999).

When employing cryo-EM the transmembrane moiety of the 16-nm plaque particles could be visualized (Oostergetel et al. 2001). Moreover, some tenuous cytoplasmic protrusions of the native AUM plaques could be directly depicted in vitrified ice that appeared as direct extensions of the six individual transmembrane domains of each plaque particle. In the investigation by Min et al. (Min et al. 2002) the 3D reconstructions of EM data recorded from negatively stained specimens confirmed the twisted ribbon-like structure of the 16 nm AUM particle at the luminal face (Fig. 4, A and B) as previously obtained by Walz, et al. (Walz et al. 1995). Mild detergent treatment, i.e. with 0.01 % triton X-100 allowed the stain to partially penetrate the membrane from the cytoplasmic side, thereby mapping out some of the plaque particle's transmembrane moiety and how it protruded into the cytoplasm, as documented in Fig. 4C.

To complement these EM-based data, I performed AFM of fully native, i.e. unfixed/ unstained urothelial plaques kept in native buffer solution. My results unveiled directly, i.e. without any image enhancement distinct protrusions of individual plaque particles on the cytoplasmic side, i.e. without any image enhancement/ or processing (Fig. 3, C and D). After averaging these particles as documented in Fig. 3E (lower part), these cytoplasmic protrusions appear as shallow, donut-shaped structures ~14 nm in diameter and ~0.5 nm in height. My results differ from those presented by Oostergetel, *et al.* (Oostergetel et al. 2001): whereas in the cryo-EM data the protrusions from the transmembrane moiety extend separately into the cytoplasm, i.e. with no contact between the individual parts of the hexameric structure, the protrusions of the urothelial plaque particles at the cytoplasmic face of the lipid membrane as depicted by AFM appeared as "closed" donut-shaped structures. Most likely, this apparent discrepancy is primarily a resolution problem caused by the movement of the cytoplasmic protrusions along the scan direction, due to the structure's softness that is stabilized when embedded in vitreous ice.

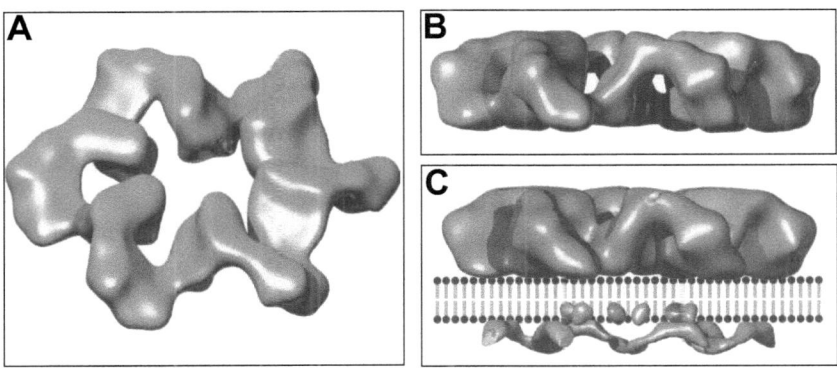

FIGURE 4: Three-dimensional reconstruction of the mouse 16 nm AUM particle as obtained by negative stain electron microscopy. (A) A 45° tilted view of a 16 nm urothelial plaque particle. (B) The side view of the AUM particle. (C) A side view of a 16 nm AUM particle in plaques that had been treated with 0.02% Triton X-100. The image visualizes the position of the lipid bilayer relative to the plaque particle. A part of the transmembrane moiety that is usually inside the bilayer became "visible" after detergent treatment, i.e. with triton X-100 and also the cytoplasmic protrusions could be visualized. The position of the lipid bilayer is simulated.

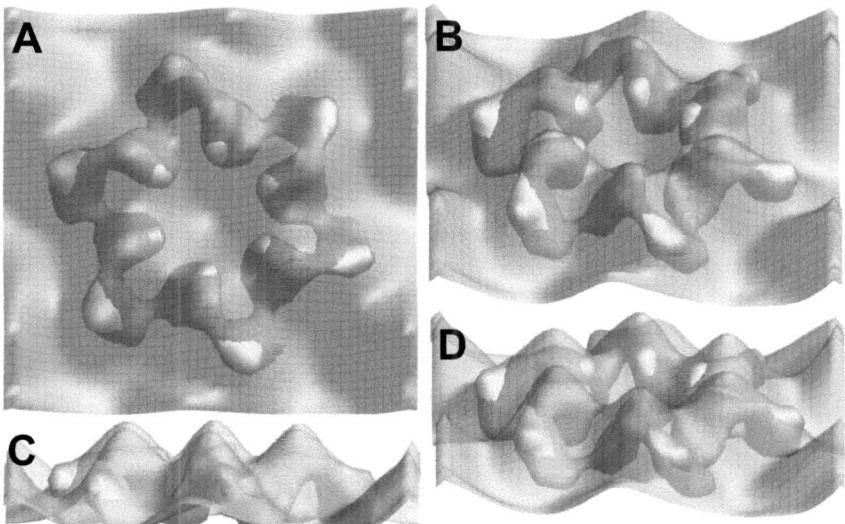

FIGURE 5: Comparison of the surface topology of urothelial 16 nm AUM particle as defined by negative staining and atomic force microscopy (AFM). The negative stained 3D reconstruction of a 16-nm mouse AUM particle (yellow) and the surface topology of a luminal urothelial plaque obtained by AFM (blue) were superimposed, and shown from the top (A), side (C) or from two other intermediate angles (B and D). For better comparison, the atomic force microscopy surface is rendered transparent and a grid mesh of the same surface is put on top of it. Note the overall consistency of the negative staining and AFM data. The negative stained particle was flatter than the AFM defined particle. This discrepancy is, particularly evident in the side view (C), most likely due to drying artifacts of the EM specimen.

In conclusion, both EM techniques, i.e. negative stain EM in combination with mild detergent treatment of the urothelial plaques and the cyo-EM data yielded similar information concerning the cytoplasmic moiety of the 16-nm plaque particle. In contrast, the AFM allowed for a direct visualization of the corrugations at the cytoplasmic surface of the urothelial plaques, i.e. without averaging or 3D reconstruction and/ or processing the raw image data. Moreover, the AFM measurements were performed in physiological buffer environment, i.e. by keeping the urothelial plaques in their native, unfixed state. Due to the high sensitivity and fidelity of recording surface corrugations of a few Å by AFM, I have been able to directly visualize the shallow, donut-like cytoplasmic moiety of the 16-nm plaque particles.

A comparison of the topology of the luminal face of AUM as visualized by AFM (Fig. 3E, upper half) versus 3D reconstructions as obtained by negative stain EM data (Fig. 4, A and B) exhibited good overall agreement of the 16-nm plaque particle. This agreement becomes even more evident when superimposing the surface topography of an AUM plaque as obtained by AFM (blue) onto the luminal 3D reconstruction of a 16 nm mouse AUM particle obtained from a negatively stained AUM plaque. As expected, the negatively stained particle was flatter than the AFM-based particle as best depicted in Fig. 5C and D. Most likely, the shallower appearance of the negatively stained 16-nm plaque particle is the consequence of drying artifacts of the specimen upon negative staining.

3.3.5 Visualization of dynamic processes: from "snap shots" to movies

3.3.5.1 Temporal resolution of dynamic biological processes at the molecular scale

A profound understanding of dynamic biological process is based on a detailed time-resolved investigation of the structural and functional aspects of the components involved. Movement or shape changes of living cells may be quite complex, but ultimately the origin of every dynamic process occurs at the level of individual biomolecules that interact with one another. Moreover, a dynamic process may involve lateral or rotational motions, as well as "spatially stationary" processes, i.e. those that do not exhibit any lateral or rotational movement like the closing and opening of gates and channels. Dynamic changes might occur at different levels of structural organization, which can be exemplified on the mammalian bladder. At the highest level this organ is a biological tissue, which is composed of cells. The cells at the bladder surface are largely covered with a biological membrane, i.e. the asymmetric unit membrane (AUM) that forms 2D crystalline patches *in situ*, called plaques. The plaques are composed of distinct 16-nm diameter particle, i.e. the urothelial plaque particles, that are hexagonally packed and based on their "folded-ribbon" topology (Walz *et al.*, (Walz et al. 1995)) are predestined to cooperatively rearrange during bladder distention. Possibly, the plaque particles might undergo a conformational change induced by some effector molecule contained in the urine. Whatever changes will be observed, a time-resolved process is of special interest.

3.3.5.2 Integrated and indirect methods for time-resolved studies

For assessing dynamic aspects of biomolecules time-resolved X-ray crystallography was employed for protein "docking" experiments in the context of designing drugs that are very sensitive to small changes being transmitted by distant effectors to eventually overcome – or compensate – a functional defect of an enzyme or receptor (Koshland 1998). Other time-resolved structural techniques are small-angle neutron or X-ray scattering, lifetime measurements of fluorophores, or stopped-flow measurements to get kinetics such as, for example, the change in concentration of the reactant and product with time. Yet another method that yields a molecular understanding of dynamic processes, such as for example, association and dissociation reactions of biomolecules, is time-resolved fluorescence spectroscopy. However, all those methods involve bulk measurement, i.e. over an area or a volume, and therefore yield an average over of the entire ensemble of a specimen rather than information on the individual molecules involved.

3.3.5.3 Direct assessment of time-resolved mechanistic processes at the level of single molecules by microscopic techniques

For most of us "seeing is believing" because the human mind can quickly grasp spatial relationships when presented in pictorial form. In contrast to spectrometers and diffractometers, microscopes allow for direct visualization of the specimen, and some microscopes even enable us to directly track biological interactions at the level of single molecules. For conducting real-time imaging, confocal laser scanning microscopy (CLSM) allows imaging of living specimens that are moving over time. However, time-resolved CLSM imaging is based on the fluorescence staining of the specimen, i.e. by fusing green fluorescent protein (GFP) to the protein(s) of interest that, in turn, may compromise the functionality of the labeled biomolecules. Moreover, this technique is dependent on the lifetime of the fluorophore and limited by a spatial resolution of ~200 nm.

As yet, the most often used microscopic technique for pursuing time-resolved structural changes of biological specimens is recording time series by cryo-EM. By this experimental approach the temporal resolution is set by the automated specimen preparation procedure employed that requires rigorous temperature and humidity control of the environment. In this approach, by aliquots of the specimen are removed at different time points and the reaction is quenched by rapid freezing of the specimen so that it becomes embedded/ surrounded by a thin film of amorphous ice suitable for static imaging by cryo-EM. By quick-freezing the sample after triggering a reaction or the start of a cycle, time-resolved "snap shots" at a resolution of ≥ 5 msec accuracy can be produced (Ruiz et al. 1994). One prominent example is the time-resolved cryo-EM analysis of microtubule dynamics, i.e. microtubule oscillation dynamic instability and turnover (Mandelkow et al. 1991).

3.3.5.4 Observation of the putative rearrangement of urothelial plaque particles while bladder distention by using time-lapse AFM

The luminal surface of the bladder epithelium provides a highly variable area that undergoes a rearrangement of the scallop shaped plaques. As yet little is known about the functional aspects of the AUM. Evidently, an assembly of single particles that are embedded in a semi-fluid lipid bilayer might interact in a cooperative manner so as to eventually yield to the formation of plaque-shaped crystalline particle arrays. Karchar *et al.* (Kachar et al. 1999) recently proposed two possible mechanisms by which AUM particles may redistribute among neighboring plaques. However any model relating to the rearrangement of single particles, formation of the inter-plaque or hinge areas and the formation of the scallop shaped plaques, so far, is rather hypothetical.

Therefore we suggest building up a device for applying mechanical stress at the whole bladder or single cells for mimicking the distortion of the bladder in its native functioning. Based on this device the AFM might then eventually allow to trace the formation, breaking up and rearrangement of whole plaques, i.e. the formation of single particles into the plaques with their crystalline package. In this scenario Fig. 3A displays a fragment of the plasma membrane with several AUM plaques that are separated by the non-crystalline hinge regions. The scallops shaped plaques with their crystalline order intersected by the hinge regions of the semifluid lipid bilayer are clearly visible. In the scenario of plaque formation or breaking up Fig. 6 could be seen as an example for a "snap shot" taken by the AFM.

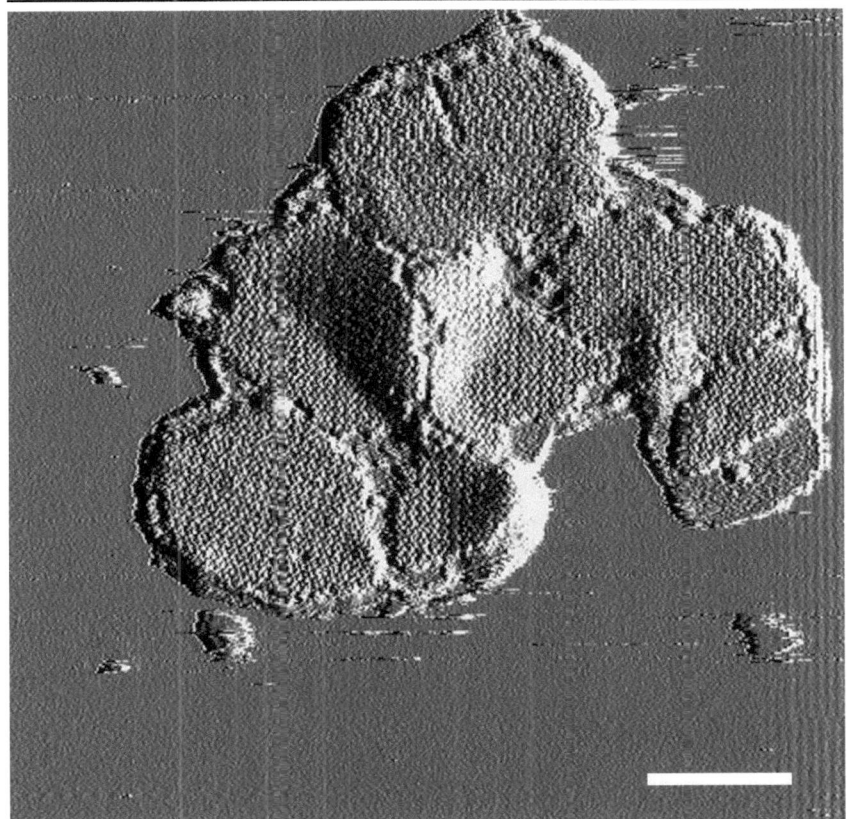

FIGURE 6: A "snap shot" of scallop shaped plaques that might have been fixed while just breaking apart or fusing and as observed by atomic force microscopy. The scallop-shaped plaques are interspersed by the hinge regions. It is proposed that in a more dynamical scenario the process of the formation of plaques potentially could be investigated by time-lapse AFM. Scale bar, 200 nm.

3.3.6 Conformational changes might occur and triggered by chemical or mechanical effectors

The AFM has the exciting possibility of potentially directly monitor structural changes at the molecular – or even submolecular scale, and directly relate these changes to biological function. As examples, height fluctuations of lysozyme molecules during substrate hydrolysis (Radmacher et al. 1994) and conformational changes in bacteriorhodopsin that are induced by increasing the loading force (Muller et al. 1997) were directly recorded by

AFM. Recently, distinct functional states of individual NPCs were recorded using time-lapse AFM (Stoffler et al. 1999).

Our AFM data have visualized the cytoplasmic domain in form of a crystalline ordering at the cytoplasmic site of the AUM. Therefore the particles protrude throughout the entire lipid bilayer. This offers the possibility that the particles may work as channels.

Currently new AFMs are designed that are specialized for a faster scanning, i.e. which allows for an up to 10 to 15-times faster recording of the data (DI, Hansma). Those developments will allow us a more close-to-real-time studying of dynamical processes.

In the context of the urothelial plaque particles, this should allow for a direct investigation of conformational changes that could be induced by chemical or mechanical effectors. With other words, the urothelial plaque particles may undergo conformational changes that could be induced by substances found in the urine, such as urea or ATP. In addition to those more chemical effectors mechanical stress or changes of the pH, such as occurring during normal bladder function potentially could also affect the structure at the level of single particles.

3.4 Conclusion

At the current stage I established a protocol for the stable immobilization of both individual faces of the AUM plaque particles in an atomic force microscope. For their imaging in a close-to-native buffer environment two distinct adsorption buffers were required, i.e. for the preferentially adsorption of the two distinct sides of AUM plaques. For high-resolution imaging a third buffer was required that balanced the tip-sample interaction for a non-destructive scanning of the protein surface. As a result, AFM of native, unfixed urothelial plaques confirmed the overall structure of the luminal 16-nm AUM particle. In addition, the overall height of the entire urothelial plaque was measured to ~12.5 nm; the height of the lipid membrane is ~5.5 nm; the leaflet above the lipid bilayer at the luminal side of urothelial plaques raised by ~6.5 nm above the luminal membrane surface. Most interestingly, AFM demonstrated for the first time donut-shaped protrusions of ~14 nm diameter and ~0.5 nm in height at the cytoplasmic side of the urothelial plaques. Next, I compared two publications with the special focus on the cytoplasmic side of the urothelial plaques. Those two publications were based on cryo-EM and negative stain EM respectively. Finally, I compared those data obtained by EM with my data obtained by AFM.

As a perspective, I proposed the functional assessment of the AUM, i.e. the investigation of a putative plaque formation but also the tracking of structural changes at the level of individual urothelial plaque particles by time-lapse AFM.

3.5 References

Aebi U, Cohn J, Buhle L, Gerace L. 1986. The nuclear lamina is a meshwork of intermediate-type filaments. *Nature* 323(6088):560-4.

Aebi U, Pollard TD. 1987. A glow discharge unit to render electron microscope grids and other surfaces hydrophilic. *J Electron Microsc Tech* 7(1):29-33.

Bremer A, Henn C, Engel A, Baumeister W, Aebi U. 1992. Has negative staining still a place in biomacromolecular electron microscopy? *Ultramicroscopy* 46(1-4):85-111.

Brisson A, Wade RH. 1983. Three-dimensional structure of luminal plasma membrane protein from urinary bladder. *J Mol Biol* 166(1):21-36.

CCP4. 1994. The ccp4 suite: Programs for protein crystallography. *Acta Cryst* D50, 760-763.

Crowther RA, Henderson R, Smith JM. 1996. Mrc image processing programs. *J Struct Biol* 116(1):9-16.

Engel A, Gaub HE, Muller DJ. 1999. Atomic force microscopy: A forceful way with single molecules. *Curr Biol* 9(4):R133-6.

Goldsbury C, Goldie K, Pellaud J, Seelig J, Frey P, Muller SA, Kistler J, Cooper GJ, Aebi U. 2000a. Amyloid fibril formation from full-length and fragments of amylin. *J Struct Biol* 130(2-3):352-62.

Goldsbury CS, Cooper GJ, Goldie KN, Muller SA, Saafi EL, Gruijters WT, Misur MP, Engel A, Aebi U, Kistler J. 1997. Polymorphic fibrillar assembly of human amylin. *J Struct Biol* 119(1):17-27.

Goldsbury CS, Wirtz S, Muller SA, Sunderji S, Wicki P, Aebi U, Frey P. 2000b. Studies on the in vitro assembly of a beta 1-40: Implications for the search for a beta fibril formation inhibitors. *J Struct Biol* 130(2-3):217-31.

Henderson R, Baldwin JM, Ceska TA, Zemlin F, Beckmann E, Downing KH. 1990. Model for the structure of bacteriorhodopsin based on high-resolution electron cryo-microscopy. *J Mol Biol* 213(4):899-929.

Hoenger A, Aebi U. 1996. 3-d reconstructions from ice-embedded and negatively stained biomacromolecular assemblies: A critiacal comparison. *J Struct Biol* 117(2):99-116.

Kachar B, Liang F, Lins U, Ding M, Wu XR, Stoffler D, Aebi U, Sun TT. 1999. Three-dimensional analysis of the 16 nm urothelial plaque particle: Luminal surface exposure, preferential head-to-head interaction, and hinge formation. *J Mol Biol* 285(2): 595-608.

Koshland DE, Jr. 1998. Conformational changes: How small is big enough? *Nat Med* 4(10):1112-4.

Lewis SA. 2000. Everything you wanted to know about the bladder epithelium but were afraid to ask. *Am J Physiol Renal Physiol* 278(6):F867-74.

Liang F, Kachar B, Ding M, Zhai Z, Wu XR, Sun TT. 1999. Urothelial hinge as a highly specialized membrane: Detergent-insolubility, urohingin association, and in vitro formation. *Differentiation* 65(1):59-69.

Mandelkow EM, Mandelkow E, Milligan RA. 1991. Microtubule dynamics and microtubule caps: A time-resolved cryo-electron microscopy study. *J Cell Biol* 114(5):977-91.

Min G, Stolz M, Zhou G, Liang F, Sebbel P, Stoffler D, Glockshuber R, Sun TT, Aebi U, Kong XP. 2002. Localization of uroplakin ia, the urothelial receptor for bacterial adhesion fimh, on the six inner domains of the 16 nm urothelial plaque particle. *J. Mol. Biol* 317(5):697-706.

Muller DJ, Schabert FA, Buldt G, Engel A. 1995. Imaging purple membranes in aqueous solutions at sub-nanometer resolution by atomic force microscopy. *Biophys J* 68(5): 1681-6.

Muller DJ, Schoenenberger CA, Schabert F, Engel A. 1997. Structural changes in native membrane proteins monitored at subnanometer resolution with the atomic force microscope: A review. *Journal of Structural Biology* 119:149-157.

Oostergetel GT, Keegstra W, Brisson A. 2001. Structure of the major membrane protein complex from urinary bladder epithelial cells by cryo-electron crystallography. *J Mol Biol* 314(2):245-52.

Radmacher M, Fritz M, Hansma HG, Hansma PK. 1994. Direct observation of enzyme activity with the atomic force microscope. *Science* 265(5178):1577-9.

Ruiz T, Erk I, Lepault J. 1994. Electron cryo-microscopy of vitrified biological specimens: Towards high spatial and temporal resolution. *Biol Cell* 80(2-3):203-10.

Schabert FA, Henn C, Engel A. 1995. Native escherichia coli ompf porin surfaces probed by atomic force microscopy. *Science* 268(5207):92-4.

Shao Z, Mou J, Czajkowsky DM, Yang J, Yuan J-Y. 1996. Biological atomic force microscopy: What is achieved and what is needed. *Advances in Physics* vol.45, no.1; Jan. Feb. 1996; p.1 86.

Stoffler D, Goldie KN, Feja B, Aebi U. 1999. Calcium-mediated structural changes of native nuclear pore complexes monitored by time-lapse atomic force microscopy. *J Mol Biol* 287(4):741-52.

Sun TT, Liang FX, Wu XR. 1999. Uroplakins as markers of urothelial differentiation. *Adv Exp Med Biol* 462:7-18.

Unwin PN. 1974. Electron microscopy of the stacked disk aggregate of tobacco mosaic virus protein. Ii. The influence of electron irradiation of the stain distribution. *J Mol Biol* 87(4):657-70.

Walz T, Haner M, Wu XR, Henn C, Engel A, Sun TT, Aebi U. 1995. Towards the molecular architecture of the asymmetric unit membrane of the mammalian urinary bladder epithelium: A closed &cuot;twisted ribbon" structure. *J Mol Biol* 248(5):887-900.

Wu XR, Manabe M, Yu J, Sun TT. 1990. Large scale purification and immunolocalization of bovine uroplakins i, ii, and iii. Molecular markers of urothelial differentiation. *J Biol Chem* 265(31):19170-9.

4. Muscle Protein Actin

4 AFM of native actin polymers and crystals after stable immobilization on supported lipid bilayers

Actin's oligomerization, polymerization, and polymorphism have been investigated over the last decade up to atomic detail by combining with X-ray and EM data. Our knowledge about actin filaments has evolved from a rigid "beads on a string model" to that of a complex, highly dynamic protein polymer (Steinmetz et al. 1997b). In contrast to electron microscopy (EM), light microscopy allows imaging of dynamic biological processes in their native aqueous environment but with a rather limited spatial resolution. As yet, the AFM is the only microscope, which can provide high resolution of biological material in its fully functional states. Thus AFM should complement our present understanding of actin filament structure, polymerization and dynamics, as well as the interaction of actin with myosin motors during muscle contraction and cell locomotion. To achieve this goal we established a protocol for stable immobilization of purified and reconstituted actin polymers and crystals on positively charged synthetic lipid bilayers. This protocol allowed us to employ AFM to image a variety of actin assemblies such as disperse filaments, paracrystalline filament arrays, and 2D crystalline sheets and tubes in physiological buffer environment. We obtained AFM data at nanometer resolution, which were compared with corresponding EM data.

4.1 Introduction

Actin plays a fundamental role in specifying cytoskeletal architecture, and it is critically involved in muscle contraction and cell motility (Schoenenberger and Hoh 1994). During muscle contraction force is generated by the cyclic interaction of the actin containing thin filaments with the myosin containing thick filaments. Changes in the mechanical properties or dynamic behavior of actin filaments are the basis for carrying out a variety of fundamental biological processes. A multitude of actin binding proteins regulates the turnover and dynamic rearrangement of the microfilament system during cell motility.

Actin is a highly conserved 43 kDa eukaryotic protein with an intrinsic ability to rapidly assemble and disassemble filamentous structures (Schoenenberger et al. 1999). At low ionic strength, purified actin is monomeric (G-actin); polymerization into filaments (F-actin) occurs when the ionic strength is raised to physiological levels (Steinmetz et al. 1997a). The combination of X-ray data obtained from G-actin with 3D reconstructions computed from electron micrographs of F-actin filaments has yielded a widely accepted atomic model for the F-actin filament. F-actin filaments are about 9 nm in diameter, and the twisted two stranded structure has a 36 nm axial crossover repeat that are assembled out of 5.5 nm sized monomers (Bremer et al. 1994). Under appropriate conditions G-actin can be induced by the trivalent lanthanide Gadolinium (Gadolinium(III) chloride hexahydrate) to form well-ordered 2D crystalline arrays including single- and double-layered sheets, and tubes (Aebi et al. 1981). The near-rectangular unit cell of the sheets, 5.6 nm x 6.5 nm, (= 87°), is a dimer with p2 symmetry. Single-layered actin sheets have an intrinsic curvature and therefore can wrap up into tubes. Alternatively, two single layered sheets can associated back-to-back to yield double-layered rectangular – or square-type sheets. Moreover, for the actin sheet terminology, architecture and polymorphism see U. Aebi, et al. (1981) (Aebi et al. 1981).

The AFM is the first instrument to record surface topographies of biological samples kept in a near-physiological environment at sub-nm resolution (Schabert et al., 1995; Müller et al. 1995a). The most exciting prospect of AFM in biology is no doubt its potential to directly monitor structural changes at the molecular – or even submolecular scale, and directly relate these changes to biological function. As examples, height fluctuations of lysozyme molecules during substrate hydrolysis were directly recorded by AFM (Radmacher et al. 1994); and conformational changes in bacteriorhodopsin that are induced by increasing the loading force (Muller et al. 1997). Recently, distinct functional states of individual NPCs were recorded using time-laps AFM (Stoffler et al. 1999).

Despite these exciting results, many important biomolecules or their supramolecular assemblies have resisted meaningful imaging by AFM in a near-physiological buffer environment. Among these are actin filaments: whereas individual actin filaments have been imaged in air and in solution by AFM, the resolution was far from molecular (Weisenhorn et al. 1990). The primary reason for this poor resolution is the fact that actin filaments cannot be stably immobilized on mica in buffer, so that they are pushed around on the substrate by the scanning tip.

When monomeric actin was applied to freshly cleaved mica, surface-induced polymerisation occurred despite buffer conditions that sustain, monomeric G-actin in solution, and a dense layer of filamentous structures was observed by AFM. The presumed F-actin was described as "blobs of 5 nm in diameter arranged in a zigzag pattern". An increase in resolution has been achieved by using tapping mode AFM (TM AFM) in liquid (Hansma et al. 1995; Moller et al. 1999; Putman et al. 1994) this imaging mode, the scanning probe is oscillated and thereby "taps" the sample (Putman et al. 1994). When imaged by TM AFM in solution, phalloidin-stabilized actin filaments, which based on the atomic model should have a diameter of 9 nm, appeared to be 20 nm high and 50 nm wide (Fritz et al. 1995). The filaments remained sufficiently stable during 10 image frames so that their 36-nm long-pitch helix crossover repeat could be resolved. In contrast to the filament width and height, this measurement is consistent with both EM and X-ray fiber diffraction data obtained from oriented F-actin gels. A similar periodicity has been measured with air-dried, phalloidin-stabilized F-actin filaments on sapphire that were fixed with glutaraldehyde prior to imaging with CMAFM (Braunstein 1995). However, the filaments observed by this approach were only ~2 nm high and ~20 nm wide. These discrepancies of filament dimensions between measurements obtained by different AFM reported using contact as well as non-contact (i.e., attractive) techniques as well as when compared with EM and X-ray diffraction data make it evident that further improvements are needed. In a recent approach F-actin was adsorbed on mica, dried in a stream of clean nitrogen gas and imaged by cryoatomic force microscopy (cryo-AFM) at liquid nitrogen temperature (Shao et al. 2000). The axial repeat has been reported with a periodicity of (38 nm and the full with at half height of (9 nm. However, a stable immobilization of actin filaments and imaging in their native environment at high resolution is still required.

4.2 Materials and Methods:

4.2.1 Materials

Unless specified otherwise, all chemicals were of analytical or best available grade. For all experiments and buffers, ultrapure deionized water was used (18 MΩ/cm; Brandstead, Boston, USA). Gadolinium(III) chloride hexahydrate, (Gadolinium) and Praseodymium(III) chloride heptahydrate (Praseodymium) was purchased from Aldrich (Aldrich, Milwaukee, Wisconsin). Phalloidin from Amanita phalloides was obtained from Sigma (Sigma, St. Louis, MO).

To prepare cationic lipid layers, the following chemicals were used: Stearylamine (SA; Sigma), 1,2-Dilauroyl-sn-Glycero-3-Phosphocholine (DLPC; Avanti Polar Lipids, Alabama, USA), Dimethyldioctadecylammonium Bromide (DDDMA; Sigma), and arachidic acid (Sigma). DDDMA-DLPC and SA-DLPC lipids were dissolved individually at ~5 mg/ml in chloroform and mixed in different ratios by volumes.

4.2.2 Actin

4.2.2.1 Preparation of actin

Rabbit skeletal muscle G-actin was prepared according to Bremer et al., (1994) at a concentration of typically 1-2 mg/ml and stored in buffer A (i.e., 2.5 mM Imidazole, pH 7.4,

0.2 mM $CaCl_2$, 0.2 mM ATP, and 0.005% NaN_3) was dialyzed at 4°C against ATP-free buffer A for 5 hours. G-actin was dialyzed into this buffer for sheets and tubes. Chemical purity of actin preparations was checked by SDS-PAGE.

To assume that a given G-actin preparation made good actin filaments and crystalline sheets, upon inducing these supramolecular assemblies, their morphology and integrity were checked by TEM of negatively stained preparations.

4.2.2.2 Preparation of F-actin paracrystals

To form F-actin filament arrays, ~30 µl polymerization buffer 50 mM KCl, 20 mM PO4, 1 mM ATP, 2 mM $MgCl_2$, pH 6.7 was pipetted into 5 x 1 mm wells in Teflon® blocks. The filled blocks were deposited onto wet filter paper kept in Petri dishes. After vortexing, ~1 µl of lipid solution, i.e. a mixture of 30:70 DDDMA-DLPC in chloroform was placed onto the buffer meniscus in each well. The chloroform was allowed to evaporate for 10-15 minutes. Meanwhile, purified rabbit skeletal muscle actin was diluted with buffer A (2.5 mM Imidazole; 0.2 mM ATP; 0.2 mM $CaCl_2$; 0.005% NaN_3) to 1 mg/ml and 0.5 µl of this G-actin solution was injected with a Hamilton syringe into the wells. To induce F-actin filament arrays, the dishes were moved to a 7 °C refrigerator for 1-2 hours, before put into a 4°C cold room for storage. Rafts were picked up with carbon-coated parlodion-films placed on 400-mesh copper grids and stored for several days to weeks to make them hydrophobic for usage in EM or with the devices described below for AFM usage.

4.2.2.3 Preparation of crystalline actin sheets and tubes

For sheet (tube) formation (Aebi et al. 1981 ; Aebi et al. 1980 ; Fowler et al. 1984; Steinmetz et al. 1998) actin was first dialyzed for 5 hrs against ATP-free buffer A at 4°C. Next the actin solution was dialyzed overnight at 4°C against 2.5 mM PIPES, pH 6.9, supplemented with 25 mM (75 mM) KCl and a 5-fold (9-fold) molar excess of Gadolinium or Praseodymium over actin.

4.2.3 Atomic force microscopy

All AFM images were recorded with a commercial TMAFM (Nanoscope III, Digital Instruments Inc., Santa Barbara, CA, USA) equipped with a 120-µm scanner (J-scanner). For high-resolution imaging, the TMAFM was placed on a bungee system for vibrational isolation. A tapping mode liquid cell without O-ring sealing was used. Prior to using, the liquid cell was carefully cleaned with a conventional dish soap, rinsed with water and then with ethanol and finally rinsed with ultrapure water. Oxide sharpened, V-shaped 100-μm long Si_3N_4 cantilevers having nominal spring constants of 0.38 N/m (Digital Instruments, Santa Barbara, CA) were used. To engage the AFM stylus, the piezo drive amplitude was set to about 170 mV. Imaging was carried out at a scan speed of 1.5 to 2 Hz. To minimize drift in the images, samples mounted for imaging were allowed to equilibrate for several minutes. All images were recorded at room temperature.

4.2.4 Electron Microscopy

For electron microscopy, 2-μl aliquots were adsorbed for 60 s to carbon-coated parlodion-films placed on 400-mesh copper grids that were previously stored for several days to weeks to make them hydrophobic. The grids were then washed for 30 s on several drops of distilled water and stained for 30 s on several drops of 0.75% uranyl formate, pH 4.25. Specimens were imaged with a Hitachi H 7000 electron microscope operated at 100 kV.

4.2.5 Immobilization of disperse F-actin filaments and of paracrystalline arrays of F-actin filaments on charged lipid monolayers starting with G-actin

Disperse F-actin filaments – or single-layered paracrystalline arrays of F-actin filaments formed by injecting G-actin into a 30-μl droplet of filament – or paracrystal-forming buffer whose surface had been coated with a positively charged lipid monolayer (30:70 DDDMA-DLPC) (Fig.1A; cf. Taylor and Taylor, 1992 (Taylor and Taylor 1992)). After 1-2 h incubation at 7°C, loose filaments (by injecting smaller amounts of G-actin) or the filament arrays that formed at the hydrophilic lipid monolayer (Fig.1B) interface were picked up with EM grids (Fig.1C, D), rinsed with polymerization buffer, negatively stained with 0.75% uranyl formate, and checked in the electron microscope (Fig. 3A, 4A). Disperse F-actin filaments and single-layered paracrystalline arrays of F-actin filaments for usage in the AFM were prepared in a similar way, i.e. by replacing the EM grid by highly oriented pyrolytic graphite (HOPG; Advanced Ceramics corp., Cleveland, OH 44107, USA) or arachidic acid coated mica followed by transferring them into the fluid cell of the AFM (Fig. 1C, D).

In more detail: When using the hydrophilic Muscovite mica (Mica New York corp., New York, NY 10013, USA) as a substrate only an even number of lipid monolayers is stable under buffer solution. Therefore a second lipid monolayer was transferred onto the hydrophobic tails of the first monolayer. In more detail, we used a) the hydrophobisation through the alkyl

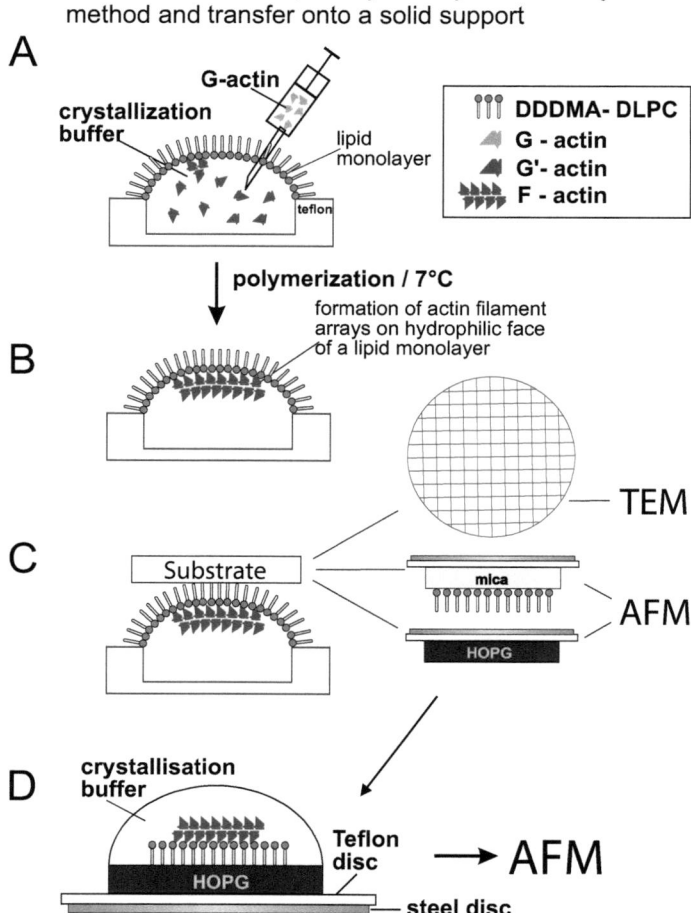

FIGURE 1: Formation of disperse actin filaments and single-layered paracrystalline actin filament arrays on a positively charged lipid monolayer consisting of a mixture of 30:70 DDDMA-DLPC, and transferred onto a solid substrate such as HOPG or mica coated with a monolayer of arachidic acid. (A) A ~30 µl drop of polymerization buffer is put into a Teflon® well onto which a 1 (l drop of the lipid mixture is spread to form a monolayer. Next, a few (l (i.e. 0.1-0.3 (l) is (typically at 1 mg/ml) injected into the buffer drop, i.e. for polymerization of disperse filaments or into single-layered paracrystalline filament arrays. (B) depending on the amount of G-actin injected and the amount of Mg^{2+} in the polymerization buffer, disperse filaments (i.e. with 2 (l actin and 0-2 mM MgCl2) or single-layered paracrystalline filament arrays (i.e. with 5 (l actin and 5-25 mM $MgCl_2$) were formed. (C) Three different solid supports, i.e. carbon-coated parlodion-films placed on 400-mesh copper grids and stored for several days to weeks to make them hydrophobic, the hydrophobic surfaces of highly oriented pyrolytic graphite (HOPG) or the hydrophobic tail-groups of arachidic acid coated mica via LB-technique were used for imaging in TEM and the latter two for usage in the AFM respectively. After 1-2 hours incubation at 7°C the monolayer was transferred onto freshly cleaved HOPG or mica coated with a lipid monolayer of arachidic acid. (D) Eventually, the specimen was put in the fluid cell of the AFM.

chains after monolayer transfer on the hydrophilic mica surface as shown in Fig. 2A or B) the hydrophobic surface of freshly cleaved HOPG (Fig. 1C) b) Small pieces (i.e. 5 x 5 mm) of the arachidic acid coated mica or the HOPG were glued with insoluble epoxy glue (Devcon, 5 minute fast drying epoxy glue, Glenview, Illinois 60025-5311, USA) onto a Teflon® disk ((~11 mm), which, in turn, had been glued with fast glue (Loctite 401, KVT Koenig AG, 8953 Dietikon, Switzerland) onto a magnetic stainless steel disk. The 2nd monolayer with the paracrystalline actin sheets was adsorbed by gently placing the so prepared sample onto the droplet (Fig. 1C). Buffer was added to avoid drying and the samples were stored at 4°C in a moist petri dish. The attachment of the filaments became more stable after (4 hours of storage. Samples were stable for at least 2 hours after mounting them in AFM. All actin filament assemblies were stabilized by stoechiometric amounts of phalloicin.

1.2.6 Immobilization of actin sheets and tubes on synthetic charged supported lipid bilayers

Muscovite mica was cut into rectangular sheets of about 3 x 4 cm and freshly cleaved with Scotch tape just before use. Arachidic acid was dissolved at 5 mg/ml in chloroform and spread onto the air/ water interface of a Fromherz Langmuir trough (P. Fromherz, Max-Planck-Institute for Biochemistry, Martinsried, Germany). The surface pressure, p, was measured with a Wilhelmy balance detecting the differential force on a piece of filter paper partially submerged in the subphase. The subphase was ultrapure water with 0.5 mM $CdCl_2$. After the chloroform evaporated for 15 minutes, the freshly cleaved mica sheets were lowered at high speed and at low p into the trough to avoid deposition of the arachidic acid onto the mica surface. The surface area was decreased to achieve a monolayer pressure of 30 mN/m, and the deposition of the lipid monolayers occurred at a speed of 2 mm/min. During this process, the monolayer pressure was held constant by electronic feedback-control of the film area (Fig. 2A).

The coated mica was cut into pieces and glued with the epoxy glue onto steel disks, which were previously cleaned with chloroform, ethanol and ultrapure water to avoid contamination of the monolayer on the LB-trough during the transfer. After some minutes of drying the mica was trimmed into the round shape of the steel disk. Two such prepared disks were held back to back by a clip and mounted on the lift. The positively charged DDDMA and neutral DLPC were mixed at different ratios and dissolved at final concentrations of 5 mg/ml in chloroform. The mixtures were spread on a subphase of ultrapure water containing 20 mM NaCl. After about 15 minutes of solvent evaporation and a deposition pressure of 40 mN/m the samples were slowly pushed down ("slow downstroke") perpendicular to the air-water interface into the trough (Fig. 2B). A second monolayer of the lipid mixture (30:

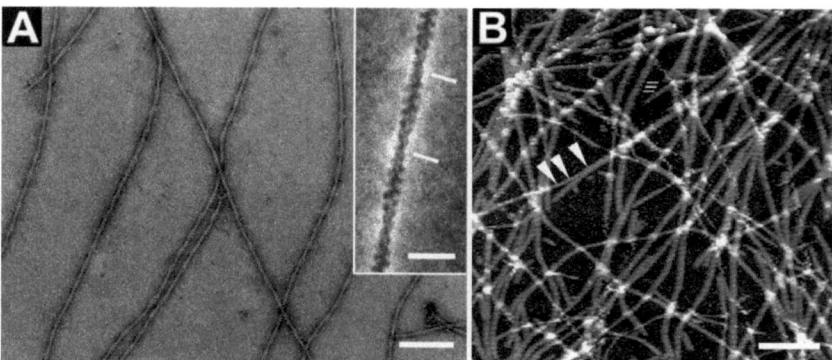

FIGURE 2: Rendering the mica surfaces via LB-technique for adsorption of actin sheets or tubes usage in AFM. (A) a monolayer of arachidic acid is transferred onto a freshly cleaved hydrophilic mica surface when the mica sheet is pulled out of the trough perpendicular through the air-water interface, i.e. via "up-stroke" (hydrophilic transfer). (B) The monolayer coated mica plate is glued onto a steel disc and two of these supports are mounted back to back by a clip. Next, a second monolayer of the mixture of 30:70 DDDMA-DLPC with its hydrophobic tail groups is transferred onto the hydrophobic tail-groups of the first monolayer of the arachidic acid via "down-stroke" (hydrophobic transfer). The net positive charge of the second transferred layer is the functional surface for adsorbing the actin sheet and tubes and is only stable under liquid. Therefore the bilayer has to be always kept under liquid. For employing the net positive charged surface for adsorbing actin sheets and tubes and then imaging in AFM a hydrophobic plastic ring is glued under water with a silicone sealant onto the supported lipid bilayer produced as shown in Fig. 2b. (C) After gluing of the plastic ring the sample then can be transferred horizontally through the air/ water interface and the water is kept onto the lipid bilayer within the inner part of the plastic ring. The sample is incubated over night and then transferred into the fluid cell of and AFM.

70 DDDMA-DLPC) is thereby transferred onto the first lipid monolayer via its hydrophobic lipid tails such that the positively charged head groups of the second monolayer are now exposed. Because the second monolayer is only stable under water and would rearrange on being retracted from water the bilayer-coated substrate was kept under water by placing it into a small plastic beaker and then transferred without exposing the bilayer to air into a bigger container for a better handling. After gluing (silicone sealant 732, Dow Corning corp., USA) a fine plastic ring (reinforcement rings, Herma GmbH, 70794 Filderstadt, Germany) onto the coated surface (Fig. 2B), the sample can be transferred horizontally through the air/ water interface to keep the water onto the lipid bilayer (Fig. 2C). Due to the hydrophobicity of this plastic ring the bilayer remains covered with water. Mounted bilayers were used on the same or next day. For the adsorption of crystalline actin sheets and tubes, the water was exchanged by slowly pipetting several times with the crystallization buffer. Next, a 5-μl aliquot of a crystalline actin sheet suspension was injected into the buffer droplet. Actin sheet and tube assemblies were stabilized by stoechiometric amounts of phalloidin. The

crystalline actin sheet and tube samples were left at 4 °C in a moist petri dish for at least 6 hours, but preferably overnight before they were transferred into the fluid cell of a Multi-Mode-AFM.

4.3 Results and Discussion

The highest resolution of biological matter has been achieved with membrane proteins adsorbed on mica surfaces (Muller et al. 1997). Immobilization of those samples is achieved by overcoming the repulsive forces by saturating the attractive forces between surface and specimen until the attractive forces become predominant (Wagner et al. 1998; Shao et al. 2000). In general, 2D crystalline protein assemblies embedded in lipid membrane patches are sufficiently stable to tolerate a wide range of pH and salt conditions so that their adsorption behavior can be optimized. In contrast, this approach has not been applicable to immobilize actin assemblies, because the structural integrity of actin polymers or crystalline arrays is very sensitive to small changes of the ion content and/ or pH of the buffer. Hence, we had to pursue another strategy, i.e. one that involved modifying the surface of the substrate in order to optimize adsorption of the actin assemblies. More specifically, we tried to optimize the right net charge, the hydrophilicity, and in addition we tried to satisfy the demand for an ultraflat surface as this is a prerequisite for high resolution by AFM.

Attempts to render the specimen support (i.e. mica) negatively or positively charged by glow discharge (Aebi and Pollard 1987) in a reduced atmosphere of air ($\rightarrow$ net negative charge) or amylamine ($\rightarrow$ net positive charge) did not yield efficient and stable adsorption of all actin samples tried. Similarly, we did not succeed to adsorb the actin assemblies onto atomically flat gold-111 surfaces, which is often used as specimen support for high resolution SPM.

Several other modifications produced a surface, which was too rough for high resolution, including the coating of mica with polylysine, which is often used to improve attachment of biomolecules to a support. Not too surprising, when we tried to coat the mica surface with a thin layer of carbon, analogous to the carbon coated EM grids used for adsorbing actin assemblies for negative stain TEM, the carbon film floated off the mica surface after getting in contact with the buffer solution.

By employing the lipid monolayer method illustrated in Fig. 1, disperse F-actin filaments and paracrystalline F-actin arrays could be adsorbed on HOPG supports (Scheuring et al. 1999). As an alternative to HOPG as just a hydrophobic support, a monolayer of arachidic acid on mica was used. Imaging of the actin assemblies adsorbed on the positive lipid layer

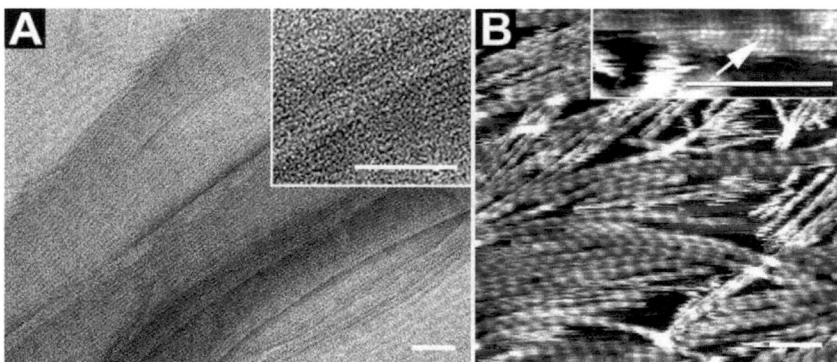

FIGURE 3: (A) Negative stain TEM image of disperse F-actin filaments grown on the positively charged surface of a lipid film (Fig.1b) before being transferred onto an EM grid (Fig.1C) and negatively stained with 0.75 % uranyl formate. (B) Disperse native actin filaments produced as described in (a) but transferred onto a hydrophobic support suitable for AFM (see Fig. 1C and D) and kept in buffer solution. AFM imaging by tapping mode of native actin filaments revealed filament dimensions (36-nm crossover repeat of the long-pitch helix crossover strand) similar to those obtained by X-ray diffraction and electron microscopy. The width is of about 40-60 nm. Scale bars: 100 nm (A); 20 nm (inset); 500 nm (B).

with arachidic acid as the supporting layer appeared a little bit more stable than the same lipid adsorbed directly onto HOPG. However, the arachidic acid film easily reorganizes into multilayers when the packing of the F-actin filaments is not very dense.

Eventually, we succeeded to stably adsorb actin assemblies onto positive charged lipid layers. The best results in terms of flatness and surface coverage were achieved by sequentially transferring two lipid monolayers onto a solid support by the LB-technique. Arachidic acid is relatively stable and yields reproducible layers of high quality and was therefore used as the first monolayer. A variety of lipids with neutral, negatively and positively charge, as well as mixtures of different ratios of these lipids were tested in view of optimizing the adsorption of the actin assemblies to the correspondingly coated supports. No or only a very weak adsorption with neutral or negatively charged surfaces was obtained. Adsorption on 30:70 DDDMA-DLPC lipid layers gave the best results also compared to the same ratio of SA-DLPC. My finding is consistent with the results obtained by Taylor & Taylor (Taylor and Taylor 1992) who found the best ordering of actin filaments by exactly these lipids and with this ratio. Other ratios of DDDMA-DLPC mixtures did not yield satisfactory adsorption.

Improved stability of filaments and crystalline sheets and tubes was observed in the presence of the bicyclic heptapeptide toxin phalloidin, which very effectively prevents the exchange of actin subunits in the actin assemblies. At the same time, tip contamination was reduced which, in turn, reduced the streaking in the fast scanning direction thereby leading to an overall enhanced resolution.

Fig. 3A reveals an electron micrograph of F-actin filaments that have been adsorbed to carbon coated film and negatively stained with uranyl formate. The inset (Fig. 3A) reveal the morphology of the actin filament, i.e. the 36 nm crossover repeat and the 5.5 nm subunits. Fig. 3B displays an AFM image of F-actin filaments produced by the monolayer method described in Fig.1, and imaged by TMAFM. Images recorded of actin filaments in tapping mode present their architecture and resolved the 36 nm crossover repeat. The filaments apperared wider, i.e. of about 40-60 nm. This is 5 to 6 times more than the expected width and can not be explained just by tip convolution. Protofilaments of amyloid that have an width of 3-5 nm appeared of about a factor of 2 wider when imaged in the AFM (Goldsbury et al. 1999). Therefore a possible explanation might be that not disperse F-actin filaments were imaged but small F-actin paracrystals of a few packed filaments.

Hoping to increase the resolution of structural detail within the filaments further, we packed the filaments into single-layered paracrystalline filament arrays were stability of individual filaments is increased by their next neighbours (Taylor and Taylor 1992). For comparison, Fig. 4A reveals a TEM micrograph of negatively stained loosely-packed single-layered paracrystalline F-actin filament arrays on a positively charged monolayer of a mixture of 30:70 DDDMA-DLPC and the corresponding sample imaged by AFM in buffer environment as illustrated in Fig. 4B. Compared to the TEM images (Fig. 4A), the AFM images reveals a better contrast due to their higher signal-to-noise ratio, and also they yield a better representation of the bona fide surface topography of the F-actin filaments. We achieved highest resolution when the fast scanning direction of the AFM was approximately parallel to the filament axis as depicted in Fig. 4B. The arrow (inset Fig. 3B) points to the (5.5 nm axial extent of individual actin subunits. In contrast to disperse actin filaments here the helicity and the 36-nm spaced axial crossover repeats of the two long-pitch helical strands of the F-actin filament are clearly visible (Steinmetz et al., 1997).

In a next step, I tried to prepare 2D crystalline actin sheets under close-to-native conditions for AFM imaging (Fig. 5). For comparison, Fig.5A displays a TEM image of a negatively stained crystalline actin sheet that had been adsorbed to a carbon-coated TEM grid.

In contrast for stable AFM imaging the actin sheets and tubes had to be adsorbed onto a supported positively charged lipid monolayer consisting of 30:70 DDDMA-DLPC in the presence of phalloidin. TMAFM imaging yielded the surface topography of the crystalline actin sheets at a resolution of about 5 nm. We also tried to prepare crystalline actin tubes for

AFM imaging. As documented in Fig. 5C, when adsorbed to a carbon-coated EM grid, the tubes spread-flatten into sheet-like structures.

In contrast, when adsorbing actin tubes to a supported lipid monolayer for AFM imaging they, at least to some extent, maintain their cylindrical shape (Fig. 5D), at the cost of resolution. We were unable to stably adsorb actin sheets and tubes in the absence of phalloidin, i.e. both conformations appeared distorted. This might be seen as an indication that phalloidin is able to stabilize sheets and tubes. Several trials to adsorb praseodymium-induced sheets onto the composite lipid films failed. The Gadolinium-induced, phalloidin stabilized sheets were the only actin assembly under investigation, for which the resolution obtained in CM AFM was equal to that in TM AFM. However, we preferred tapping mode because it reduced tip contamination compared to contact mode.

Adsorption of actin sheets and tubes onto (pre-) formed lipid bilayers

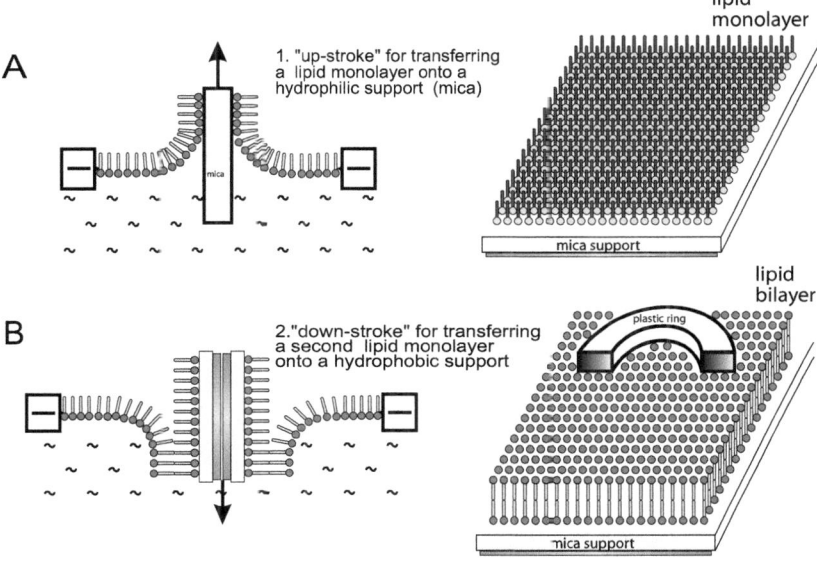

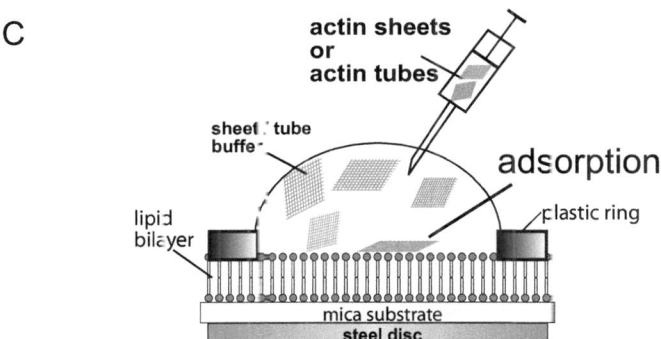

FIGURE 4: Formation of single-layered paracrystalline actin filament arrays on a positively charged monolayer of a mixture of 30:70 DDDMA-DLPC (see Fig. 1) and imaged by TEM or AFM. (A) TEM image of negatively stained (i.e., with 0,75% uranyl formate, pH 4.25) single-layered paracrystalline actin filament arrays. (B) Tapping mode image of native single-layered paracrystalline actin filament arrays kept in buffer solution exhibiting the 36-nm crossover spacing of the two long-pitch helical strands within the individual actin filaments. Higher magnification images of an actin filament as shown in the inset (B) reveal the 5.5-nm axial repeat of the actin subunits within individual filaments. Scale bars: 500 nm (A); 200 nm (inset); 100 nm (B); and 100 nm (inset).

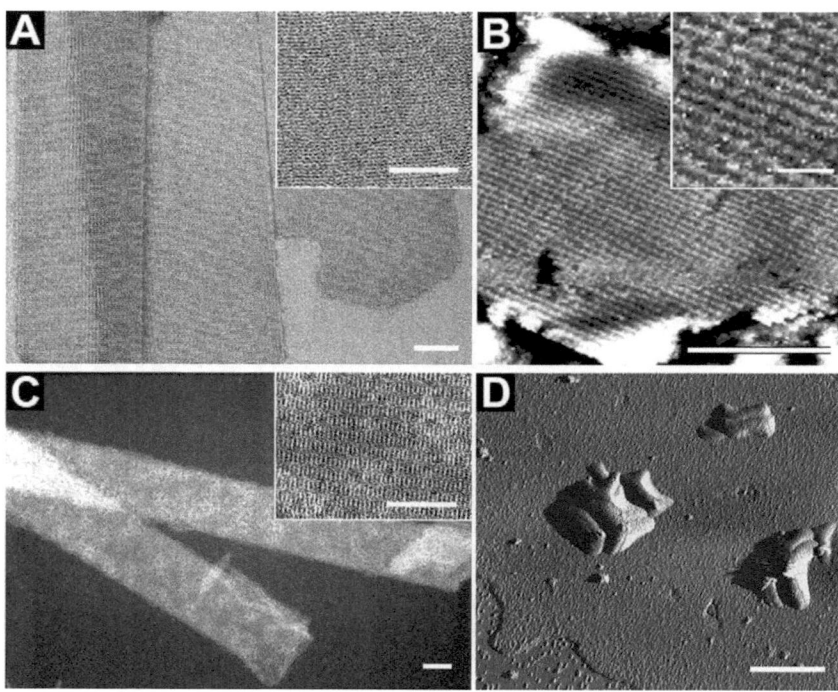

FIGURE 5: (A, C) EM and (B, D) AFM imaging by tapping mode of native double-layered crystalline actin sheets and tubes which have been immobilized on the positively charged surface of a mica-supported lipid bilayer and kept in buffer solution. Tapping mode AFM imaging of native actin sheets and tubes kept in crystallization buffer. The sheet shown in (B) reveals distinct rows of actin dimers. The spacing between rows is (5.6 nm. In the higher magnification inset in (B) individual actin subunits can be depicted in places that are spaced by about 3.3 nm along the distinct rows. As documented in Fig. 5C, when adsorbed to a carbon-coated EM grid, the tubes spread-flatten into sheet-like structures. In contrast, actin tubes repaired for AFM appear cylindrical when imaged in by TMAFM (Fig. 5D). All scale bars, 100 nm, except inset in 5B, 20 nm, 5D, 500 nm.

4.4 Conclusions

Two methods were employed to achieve direct adsorption of actin assemblies onto high-quality supported synthetic lipid bilayers: (i) the lipid monolayer method for immobilizing F-actin filament arrays that were directly grown onto the lipid monolayer and then transferred onto a hydrophobic supported surface and (ii) native double-layered crystalline actin sheets and tubes which have been previously synthesized in a test tube and then immobilized on the positively charged surface of a mica-supported lipid bilayer. For both methods the use of a mixture of net positively charged lipids (30:70 DDDMA-DLPC) has yielded stable immobilization of the native actin assemblies on solid supports suitable for high-resolution AFM imaging.

In more detail, F-actin filament arrays were directly grown onto the positive charged lipid layer at the air-water interface of a droplet sitting in Teflon® well (see Fig. 1A and B). The situation on the surface of the droplet is similar to that on the air/water interface of a LB-trough such that in both techniques the lipid monolayer is unsupported, i.e. at the air-water interface. However, on the droplet the lateral surface pressure of the lipid film is determined by the curvature or the size of the droplet and can not further be controlled as this is done by the feedback controlled barriers in a LB-trough. After injection of the G-actin and polymerization onto the lipid monolayer (Fig. 1A and B) the paracrystalline actin filament arrays are then picked up for immobilization onto a hydrophobic support, i.e. on hydrophobic EM grids, HOPG or monolayer coated mica and then transferred into the EM or AFM for imaging (see Fig. 1C and D). Compared to disperse actin filaments (or possibly small F-actin paracrystals of a few packed filaments) the formation of single-layered paracrystalline actin filament arrays revealed not only the 36 nm crossover repeat but also the 5.5 nm subunits. This might be seen as a conformation of the thesis that soft biological matter can best be imaged, i.e. with sub-molecular resolution by AFM by employing well ordered periodic specimens at best 2D crystals.

The second method is the LB-technique that produces a lipid bilayer coated mica support (see Fig. 2). Onto those ulraflat and net positively charged surface crystalline actin sheets and tubes were deposited. Here the specimens are well ordered periodic specimens. Similarly, AFM images of crystalline actin sheets recorded in tapping mode depicted the packing of the actin dimers within their near-rectangular, 5.6 nm x 6.5 nm unit cell.

As a result of these improvements in specimen preparation we eventually succeeded to reproducibly image actin in its native state. The contrast and signal-to-noise ratio of these AFM images was good enough that actin assemblies could be directly, i.e. without major image processing compared and correlated with corresponding EM images. Since the AFM allows imaging the 3D topography the imaging also gives information in the third dimension.

Most of the presently available structural information represents actin in one specific functional state. We have been trying to image actin filaments by AFM in their native state and directly determine the surface topography of the two faces of crystalline actin crystalline actin sheets or G-actin tubes under native conditions by AFM, a) to compare the native structure of the filament with its atomic model, but also b) to eventually directly monitor structural changes induced by chemical or mechanical effectors.

We are confident that by optimizing both sample preparation and imaging, we may ultimately achieve a resolution of about 2 nm with actin filament arrays and about 1 nm with crystalline actin arrays. This, obviously, is a prerequisite for investigating some of the more dynamic aspects of the actin filament such as its subtle structural – and in turn mechanical – changes occurring in response to a variety of physiological effectors, ligands and interacting proteins (cf. Steinmetz et al., (Steinmetz et al. 1997a; Steinmetz et al. 1997b))

4.5 References

Aebi U, Fowler WE, Isenberg G, Pollard TD, Smith PR. 1981. Crystalline actin sheets: Their structure and polymorphism. *J Cell Biol* 91(2 Pt 1):340-51.

Aebi U, Pollard TD. 1987. A glow discharge unit to render electron microscope grids and other surfaces hydrophilic. *J Electron Microsc Tech* 7(1):29-33.

Aebi U, Smith PR, Isenberg G, Pollard TD. 1980. Structure of crystalline actin sheets. *Nature* 288(5788):296-8.

Braunstein D. 1995. Imaging an f-actin structure with noncontact scanning force microscopy. *J. Vac. Sci. Technol. A* 13 (3):1733-1736.

Bremer A, Henn C, Goldie KN, Engel A, Smith PR, Aebi U. 1994. Towards atomic interpretation of f-actin filament three-dimensional reconstructions. *J Mol Biol* 242(5): 683-700.

Fowler WE, Buhle EL, Aebi U. 1984. Tubular arrays of the actin-dnase i complex induced by gadolinium. *Proc Natl Acad Sci U S A* 81(6):1669-73.

Fritz M, Radmacher M, Cleveland JP, Allersma MW, Stewart RJ, Gieselmann R, Janmey P, Schmidt CF, Hansma PK. 1995. Imaging globular and filamentous proteins in physiological buffer solutions with tapping mode atomic force microscopy. *Langmuir* 11:3529-3235.

Goldsbury C, Kistler J, Aebi U, Arvinte T, Cooper GJ. 1999. Watching amyloid fibrils grow by time-lapse atomic force microscopy. *J Mol Biol* 285(1):33-9.

Hansma HG, Laney DE, Bezanilla M, Sinsheimer RL, Hansma PK. 1995. Applications for atomic force microscopy of DNA. *Biophys J* 68(5):1672-7.

Moller C, Allen M, Elings V, Engel A, Muller DJ. 1999. Tapping-mode atomic force microscopy produces faithful high-resolution images of protein surfaces. *Biophys J* 77(2):1150-8.

Muller DJ, Schoenenberger CA, Schabert F, Engel A. 1997. Structural changes in native membrane proteins monitored at subnanometer resolution with the atomic force microscope: A review. *Journal of Structural Biology* 119:149-157.

Putman CAJ, van dWKO, de GBG, van HNF. 1994. Tapping mode atomic force microscopy in liquid. *Applied Physics Letters* vol.64, no.18; 2 May 1994; p.2454 6.

Radmacher M, Fritz M, Hansma HG, Hansma PK. 1994. Direct observation of enzyme activity with the atomic force microscope. *Science* 265(5178):1577-9.

Scheuring S, Muller DJ, Ringler P, Heymann JB, Engel A. 1999. Imaging streptavidin 2d crystals on biotinylated lipid monolayers at high resolution with the atomic force microscope. *Journal of Microscopy* 193(1):28-35.

Schoenenberger CA, Hoh JH. 1994. Slow cellular dynamics in mdck and r5 cells monitored by time-lapse atomic force microscopy. *Biophys J* 67(2):929-36.

Schoenenberger CA, Steinmetz MO, Stoffler D, Mandinova A, Aebi U. 1999. Structure, assembly, and dynamics of actin filaments in situ and in vitro. *Microsc Res Tech* 47(1):38-50.

Shao Z, Shi D, Somlyo AV. 2000. Cryoatomic force microscopy of filamentous actin. *Biophys J* 78(2):950-8.

Steinmetz MO, Goldie KN, Aebi U. 1997a. A correlative analysis of actin filament assembly, structure, and dynamics. *J Cell Biol* 138(3):559-74.

Steinmetz MO, Hoenger A, Tittmann P, Fuchs KH, Gross H, Aebi U. 1998. An atomic model of crystalline actin tubes: Combining electron microscopy with x-ray crystallography. *J Mol Biol* 278(4):703-11.

Steinmetz MO, Stoffler D, Hoenger A, Bremer A, Aebi U. 1997b. Actin: From cell biology to atomic detail. *J Struct Biol* 119(3):295-320.

Stoffler D, Goldie KN, Feja B, Aebi U. 1999. Calcium-mediated structural changes of native nuclear pore complexes monitored by time-lapse atomic force microscopy. *J Mol Biol* 287(4):741-52.

Taylor KA, Taylor DW. 1992. Formation of 2-d paracrystals of f-actin on phospholipid layers mixed with quaternary ammonium surfactants. *J Struct Biol* 108(2):140-7.

Wagner P. 1998. Immobilization strategies for biological scanning probe microscopy. *FEBS Lett* 430(1-2):112-5.

Weisenhorn AL, Drake B, Prater CB, Gould SA, Hansma PK, Ohnesorge F, Egger M, Heyn SP, Gaub HE. 1990. Immobilized proteins in buffer imaged at molecular resolution by atomic force microscopy. *Biophys J* 58(5):1251-8.

5. Indentation Testing of Soft Biological Tissues

5 Assessing the biomechanical properties of normal, diseased and engineered tissue by indentation-type atomic force microscopy

Well-established indentation testing procedures are available for determination of a material's mechanical properties (e.g., stiffness and strength). Those indentation tests were originally developed in the material sciences for measuring the mechanical properties of hard solids, e.g., ceramics and metals, but are more frequently used for testing of soft biological tissues. In the context of life science, the AFM is capable of imaging, measuring and manipulating biological tissues, such as cartilage, bone and blood vessels under physiological buffer conditions. The fundamental processes in biology and especially of tissue degeneration are occurring at the molecular scale where the AFM provides far greater dimensional sensitivity compared to conventional clinical indentation testing devices for mechanical testing of small samples. This potentially opens new vistas for obtaining additional wealth of information when assessing the biomechanical properties at smaller scales as this is currently done. AFM-based technology bears the promise to assess the mechanical properties starting from the level of proteins to living cells up to the complex network of a whole tissue, i.e. at all relevant levels of tissue's hierarchic structural organization, first *ex vivo* and ultimately *in situ*.

More specifically, IT AFM which is based on piezoelectric actuators has far greater dimensional sensitivity compared to conventional clinical indentation testing devices. This technical improvement compared to, for example, mechanical indentation testing devices allows for higher-resolution indentation testing data and therefore suggests that IT AFM can be used to explore and better understand the effects of disease, injury and treatment on soft biological tissue, and perhaps detect early changes in a disease. To explore and validate the practical use of IT AFM, we are currently focusing on two frequent and devastating diseases, i.e. osteoarthritis and arteriosclerosis. Ultimately, we want to move IT AFM from the bench to the patient by directly bringing the AFM to the disease site *via* an endoscopic approach.

5.1 Assessing the mechanical properties of porcine cartilage tissue at the nanometer and micrometer scale by indentation-type atomic force microscopy

Compared to hard solids, such as metals, ceramics and polymers, biological tissues typically possess much more complex and hierarchic structures, comprised of a variety of solid and liquid phase components (Cohen et al. 1998; Lai et al. 1991; Mow et al. 1980). Articular cartilage is employed as a prime example of a complex tissue material of varying composition. Its major function is the protection of the joint surfaces and the transduction of forces through the joints. Within the tissue a relative small amount of chondrocytes, i.e. the cartilage cells express a complex network called the extracellular matrix (ECM). The ECM is comprised of (i) a cross-linked network of ~50 nm diameter type II collagen fibers (10-20 wt. %), interspersed with, but not bonded to (ii) proteoglycan aggregates (long-chain ~10^6 kDa hyaluronate glycosaminoglycan molecules to which shorter-chain sulfated glycosaminoglycan molecules are attached) (4-7 wt. %), and (iii) water (65-80 wt. %). Biochemical and structural alterations as they are occurring in pathological situations such as trauma or chronic tissue damage (e.g., osteoarthritis) may have a direct impact of the functional performance of native and diseased cartilage tissue. However, under loading pressure the bound water is moved through the porous-like matrix. Consequently, with increasing time of loading when resting in a musculo-skeletal position, e.g. while waiting for the bus, the pure elastical properties of the cartilage tissue get dominated by time-dependent viscoelastic effects (Cohen et al. 1998). However, from a more practical point of view the short-term biomechanical functionality of articular cartilage is of primary interest as it occurs while walking, running or jumping. For example, the loading of a human knee joint while jumping, running or marching takes some tens to some hundreds milliseconds (Popko et al. 1986) and thus may be most sensitively characterized by measuring the elastical properties of the cartilage tissue.

The most comprehensive information about the functioning or mal-functioning of articular cartilage tissue can be obtained by measuring its biomechanical properties (Armstrong and Mow 1982; Cohen et al. 1998; Roth and Mow 1980). In the context of assessing the biomechanical properties of articular cartilage tissue, IT AFM offers to characterize and control pathological changes at an early stage of the disease progression when it's still reversible.

5.2 Relevance of elasticity measurements of articular cartilage tissue by indentation-type AFM

Pathological situations such as acute trauma or chronic tissue damage potentially lead to the depletion of the articulating surfaces in joints, such as the knee and hip (McDevitt and Muir 1976). The regeneration or repair of diseased articular cartilage can be stimulated by growth factors or other therapeutical approaches (Polisson 2001; Van den Berg et al. 2001). At a more advanced state eventually the defect has to be repaired by orthopedic surgery were some of the diseased tissue has to be replaced by transplants. Cartilage plaques for joint replacement can be harvested from non-load bearing parts in the form of autografts that were taken from the same organism or by allografts from foreign tissue. Unfortunately, the amount of autografts is naturally limited. Moreover, when transplanting allografts unforeseen adverse effects caused by autoimmune responses or infectious diseases such as hepatitis and HIV/AIDS might be minimized but cannot be excluded. Hence, the creation of artificial cartilage by tissue engineering approaches holds promise for direct implantation in the articular joint disease site.

Whatever might be the particular strategy for the individual patient, this load-bearing native or artificial articular cartilage must be mechanically functional (Ma et al. 1995). To date the success of therapeutic approaches or transplantation still is often tested by the well-being of the patient a long time after the surgery. This represents a rather subjective way and requires a more objective method of testing the quality of the patient's joint properties. Moreover, the functionality of the articulating surface and the durability of the implant should best be measured before and after the surgery. Quantitative analysis to detect cartilage functionality or pathological alterations to date are most frequently provided by imaging techniques, e.g. X-ray transmission imaging (X-ray), computed topography (CT) and by magnetic resonance imaging (MRI) but also by arthroscopical techniques. Those imaging methods can resolve structural details, and provide biomechanical properties of the tissue but generally reveal notable changes at a significant advanced state of degradation, including tissue erosion, which are essentially irreversible. In contrast, deformation-based techniques relate directly to the mechanical properties of the underlying tissue. However, clinical indenters typically employ indenter sizes at the millimeter scale (Appleyard et al. 2001; Aspden et al. 1991; Lyyra et al. 1999; Shepherd and Seedhom 1997), i.e. of the same range as the thickness of most of the tissues to be measured. Elasticity values gathered with such devices may thus rather relate to that of the supporting substrate, especially in small joints, where cartilage layers are thin. In any case, these methods are not sensitive enough to pick up changes of a disease progression especially at an early state of a disease.

In a first example, I want to provide measurements of cartilage elasticity similar as those obtained by clinical indentation testing devices. This involves the deduction of the elastic modulus from the unloading load-indentation curve. In the following chapter I'm shortly giving a definition of hardness measurements and the elastic modulus. I want to put special emphasis in the conduction of these two parameters and how they can be derived from indentation curves.

5.2.1 Methods used for characterization of mechanical properties

5.2.1.1 Hardness

Hardness is the classical parameter for characterizing the mechanical robustness of a load bearing surface. Typical applications for hardness measurements are high quality tools, ball bearings or implants for hip replacement.

When performing a hardness measurement, an indenter with a precisely defined shape is driven uniaxially into the surface of the specimen surface with a given maximum load. According to its conventional definition the hardness value is calculated by dividing its maximal load through the projected area of the permanent indent. For the analysis, the permanent indent can be measured by microscopically techniques, such as SEM, TEM or AFM. In contrast to this more conventional hardness measurement procedure to date indentation testing typically is based on fully computerized instruments that allow for a continuous recording of the entire loading and unloading cycle while the indenter is pushed into and retracted from the surface. This allows for the calculation of the projected area as a function of the displacement of the tip and the applied load during the entire indentation process in space and time. Hardness is defined as the maximal load divided by the projected area[3] at maximum load and, i.e. in contrast to the projected area of the permanent indent.

---

[3] The projected area is **not** identical to the geometry of the indenter. (If a finger is pressed into a drum the indent is larger than the shape of the finger tip.) The corresponding projected area is calculated by the underlying model, i.e. Hertz, Sneddon, Oliver & Pharr, whereas the classical Hertzian model accounts only for the contact of two half spheres (or the indent of a half sphere into a half space = sphere with an infinite radius of curvature). Sneddon expanded the Herzian theory to the indenter shapes mentioned below; and Oliver and Pharr refined the model to materials with non-ideal elastic behavior.

When performing a hardness measurement the following aspects are of special interest: (1) A hardness measurement is always based on the analysis of the **loading** curve that accounts for numerous non-elastic properties of the sample, such as plasticity and viscoelasticity. (2) The loading curve accounts for the shape of the indenter, i.e. the loading data include parameters specified by the instrumental setup. Hence, hardness is not simply a material parameter, but it also depends on the particular instrumental setup used for the measurement.

Next, I want to briefly describe some of the frequently employed indenters used for performing hardness measurements on solid-state specimens and biomaterials:

- **Vickers indenter:** a four-sided symmetrical pyramid with an exactly defined centerline-to-face angle. The tip of the 4-sided pyramid, rather being point-like, typically exhibits a "chisel-edge" shape.

- **Berkovich indenter:** a three-sided pyramid that can be readily ground into a point and hence is the commonly used indenter shape used for microhardness testing.

- **Spherical indenter:** while pressing a spherical indenter into a planar surface a point contact is first encountered that in the absence of sharp corners and edges, produces only linear elastic deformations that can readily be modeled. Hence, the spherical indenter appears to be ideally suited for the applications that are the focus of my thesis. Unfortunately, it is rather difficult to manufacture a spherical indenter shape at the sub-micrometer scale.

- **Flat-punch indenter:** This cylindrical indenter has a sharp ring-like rimp. In contrast to a spherical indenter it is much more difficult to position this indenter perpendicular to the surface and in addition to provide an uniaxial indentation.

Vickers-like indenters are etched along the crystalline faces of the silicon. Vickers and Berkovich indenters can be produced with high precision at small scales and therefore are typically used for AFM. As the hardness value for a given material depends on the indenter used for the measurement, this should always be specified, e.g. Vickers hardness.

5.2.1.2 Elastic modulus

The measurement of the elastic modulus should always be based on the analysis of the **unloading** load indentation-curve. While the loading curve might include non-elastical contributions, i.e. mainly plasticity, the unloading curve ideally reflects only the pure linear elastic material response to the indentation process applied to the sample. However, this is only true over a relatively short time scale, where the term "relative" depends on the material, in particular, its viscoelastic properties. Moreover, it assumes that the loading exerted a linear elastic deformation, i.e. a deformation that did not generate an elastical flow during indentation. To achieve a linear elastic deformation an appropriate loading rate has to be chosen for yielding faithful elasticity data.

Unlike the hardness (see above), the elastic modulus is a **material constant**, i.e. it is independent of the shape of the indenter. However, the difficulty for analyzing the unloading load-displacement curves is to precisely model the course of the projected area during unloading[4]. The underlying model, i.e. usually in the form of a mathematical equation, describes the time-dependent shape of the recorded unloading curve with the elastic modulus representing one important physical material parameter. The second essential parameter is the so-called shape factor of the indenter: i.e. when taking a "snapshot" at a given time point during the unloading phase the precise projected area and the corresponding load acting on the indenter can thus be determined. The load is then simply given by Hook's law.

Mechanical properties of cartilage.

Because of its composition and structure, cartilage behaves mechanically as a viscoelastic solid. Therefore, its mechanical properties (e.g., stiffness, strength) depend on the rate of strain or the rate of stress depending on which parameter is controlled. Also, under cyclic loading, the applied stress and the resulting strain are not in phase. For compressive or tensile strains, the ratio of stress to strain in this case is the dynamic elastic modulus, $|E^*|$, which is the vector sum of the storage modulus E' (the in-phase, elastic component) and the loss modulus E" (the out-of-phase, viscous component). In contrast, for solid materials that behave elastically (e.g., steel), cyclic stress and strain are in phase, i.e., no energy

---

[4] The time-dependent change of the projected area as reflected in the load-indentation curve is described by a mathematical equation. For obtaining good data the tip has to be placed exactly perpendicular to the sample surface to provide an indent in direction of the axis of the indenter. Any torsion of the cantilever causes a "distortion" in the load-indentation curve and hence a deviation from the mathematical ideal shape as imposed by the underlying model.

dissipation occurs in the elastic range and all applied energy is stored, not lost, and the ratio of stress to strain is the elastic modulus, E (also having units of force/area). The general term, "stiffness", is used to describe the relation between stress and strain determined under various loading modes below the stress level which causes permanent deformation. In tension and compression, the quantities are E and $|E^*|$ as described, whereas in shear, the analogous quantities are G and $|G^*|$.

For clarification, the shear modulus G and the extensional modulus E are related for homogenous, isotropic materials by $E = 2G (1 + v)$, where v is Poisson's ratio, so for $v = 0.5$, $E = 3 G$. The indentation modulus is usually an extensional modulus, E, although the state of stress is actually a mixture of compression and shear, mainly. In the work presented here an indentation modulus, E, with the microspherical probe and a modulus value from the calibration curve based on compression elastic modulus, E, was measured (see Materials and Methods). Because the measurements presented here are dynamic, the use of $|E^*|$ in place of E is appropriate, and for the materials presented here, with $v = 0.5$, it should be appropriate to assume that $|E^*| = 3 |G^*|$ so the measurements can be related to the results of Mankin.

5.2.1.3 Indentation testing device resolution capability

For accurate determination of the stiffness of a sample, its mechanical response should be independent of the mechanical property response of the underlying substrate or support. According to the rule of Bueckle (Bueckle 1973; Persch et al. 1994), the depth of indentation should therefore be not more than 10% of the sample thickness. Because most biological specimens are limited in their size, only small indentation depths are possible. For example, the thickness of cartilage covering the articulating surfaces of human joints is typically 1-4 mm (Swanepoel et al. 1994) and consequently the maximal indentation depth is between 0.1 and 0.4 mm. To achieve such small indentation depths, high resolution monitoring of the z-displacement of the indenter is required.

The accuracy of the z-displacement can be characterized by the signal-to-quantization-noise ratio (SQNR), which is the ratio between the z-displacement signal in the load-displacement curve and the noise due to the approximation or quantization error in the z-position of the indenter. Clinical indentation testing devices typically have a z-position resolution of about ± 10 µm (Aspden et al. 1991). Thus, the true z-position values are within intervals of ± 10 µm and are assumed to be Gaussian distributed (Lueke 1992). When employing such a clinical testing device for testing articular cartilage (assuming a 4 mm thickness), optimally N = 40 sample points can be taken over the whole range of indentation, i.e. 0.4 mm, while recording a single loading/ unloading data set. Then the SQNR can be calculated (Lueke 1992):

(1) $SQNR \approx N \times 6dB$; N is an integer number to quantify the system;

(2) $N \geq lb \times (h_{max}/\Delta)$

lb = logarithm to basis 2, h_{max} = maximal depth of indentation, Δ = z-positioning accuracy of the indentation device, i.e. its z-positioning error.

For such a clinical indentation testing device with a z-positioning accuracy of $\pm$ 10 μm one obtains a $SQNR_{clinic}$ of $\approx$36 dB. A similar calculation of the SQNR for IT AFM that has a z-positioning accuracy of $\pm$ 0.1 nm (Hues et al. 1993), results to $SQNR_{AFM} \approx$132 dB. Because a specific indentation testing device has a limited and fixed z-resolution capability, Δ, a higher SQNR thus can only be obtained by increasing the depth of indentation, h_{max}, which then increases the number of sample points N (see Equation 1). However, an increase of the depth of indentation then violates the rule of Bueckle.

5.2.1.4 Corollaries

- Many of the published elastic moduli of biological tissues have been determined by analyzing the loading curves of the indenters employed. For very elastic tissues (i.e. soft tissues) the error might be negligible. In fact, biological tissues exhibit significant plasticity and/ or viscoelasticity so that the analysis of their loading curves yields false elasticity values.

- By determining a physically well-defined material parameter, i.e. the elastic modulus, its measurement should be device-independent. This is an important prerequisite when trying to establish a reference database that is meant to faithfully represent the relative elastic properties of different articular cartilage, i.e. normal versus diseased or engineered cartilage.

- Articular cartilage tissue exhibits a distinct viscoelastic behavior: While waiting for a bus in an inert musculo-skeletal position, its entire synovial fluid of, let's say the articular cartilage has enough time to be squeezed through the sponge-like extracellular matrix. In contrast, at a shorter time scale less synovial fluid is moved through the tissue and therefore the articular cartilage's elastic properties are dominating viscoelastical properties. As a consequence, all elasticity data determined in the course of this thesis are based on three complete loading/ unloading cycles per second, i.e. at 3 Hz. This are typically much faster unloading times compared to testing protocols of hard solids and therefore I'm more appropriately using the term, dynamic elastic modulus. Hence, each unloading time corresponds to ~150 ms. This are typical physiological loading/ unloading times as they are encountered by our knee joints while walking, running or jumping, so that the dynamic elastic properties of the articular knee cartilage should well predominate over its viscoelastic properties

The method described in the following sections has been mainly developed on amorphous agarose gels and on (structured) articular cartilage tissue. However, this method should be also applicable for the measurement of the elastic moduli of other biological tissues.

5.3 Dynamic elastic modulus of articular cartilage determined at two different levels of tissue organization by indentation-type atomic force microscopy

Cartilage stiffness was measured *ex vivo* at the micrometer and nanometer scale (Table 1) to explore structure-mechanical property relationships at smaller scales than has been done previously. A method was developed to measure the dynamic elastic modulus, $|E^*|$, in compression by indentation-type atomic force microscopy (IT AFM). Spherical indenter tips (radius ~2.5 µm) and sharp pyramidal tips (radius ~20 nm) were employed to probe micrometer-scale and nanometer-scale response, respectively. $|E^*|$ values were obtained at 3 Hz from 1,024 unloading response curves recorded at a given location on sub-surface cartilage from porcine femoral condyles. With the microsphere tips, the average modulus was ~2.6 MPa, in agreement with available millimeter-scale data, whereas with the sharp pyramidal tips, it was typically 100-fold lower. In contrast to cartilage, measurements made on agarose gels, a much more molecularly amorphous biomaterial, resulted in the same average modulus for both indentation tips. From results of AFM imaging of cartilage, the micrometer scale spherical tips resolved no fine structure except some chondrocytes, while the nanometer scale pyramidal tips resolved individual collagen fibers and their 67 nm axial repeat distance. These results suggest that the spherical AFM tip is large enough to measure the aggregate dynamic elastic modulus of cartilage, whereas the sharp AFM tip depicts the elastic properties of its fine structure. Additional measurements of cartilage stiffness following enzyme action revealed that elastase digestion of the collagen moiety lowered the modulus at the micrometer scale. In contrast, digestion of the proteoglycans moiety by

	nano-regime	**micro-regime**
radius of the tip	several nanometers (i.e. ~ 20 nm)	few micrometers (i.e. ~ 2.5 μm)
applied load	nanonewton (i.e. ~ 1.8 nN)	micronewton (i.e. 15 nN - 3.3 μN)
indentation depth	several 10 to a few 100 nanometers (i.e. 300 - 550 nm)	several 100 nanometers (i.e. 250 - 600 nm)

TABLE 1: Comparison of test parameters between the nanometer or micrometer scale modulus measurements of soft biological materials by IT AFM.

cathepsin D had little effect on $|E^*|$ at the micrometer scale, but yielded a clear stiffening at the nanometer scale. Thus, cartilage compressive stiffness is different at the nanometer scale compared to the overall structural stiffness measured at the micrometer and larger scales because of the fine nanometer-scale structure, and enzyme-induced structural changes can affect this scale-dependent stiffness differently.

5.4 Introduction

Stiffness is the mechanical parameter describing the relation between an applied, non-destructive load and resultant deformation of a material. It can be determined at all scales of a material's internal structure, and will vary if the measuring device addresses different structural elements rather than their aggregation. It also often varies with the nature of the load (e.g. tension, compression, and shear), the rate of deformation, and whether deformation is monotonic or cyclic.

Additionally, stiffness can be sensitive to the internal structural details of heterogeneous materials and thus can be used as a probe of hierarchical structure-property relationships. A large body of data is available describing the compressive stiffness of articular cartilage at the millimeter scale. These stiffness values have often been measured *in situ* by indentation testing using clinical millimeter-scale indentation devices during arthroscopic surgery. The purpose of such studies is to help surgeons assess and map the load-bearing capacity or "health" of the cartilage, and to better understand how cartilage pathology affects this key mechanical property.

Two mechanisms are responsible for the viscoelastic behavior of cartilage: (i) a flow-independent mechanism, intermolecular friction, exhibited in all polymeric materials, and (ii) a flow-dependent mechanism that is present if loading conditions allow water to move through the structure. However, in ambulation (i.e. walking, running), loading and unloading are transient events, occurring in < 1 second. Under these conditions, essentially no motion of water through the structure occurs, due to the high drag coefficient ($\sim 10^{14}$ Ns/m^4, Mankin et al. 1994). Hence, the mechanical response of cartilage should be measured under dynamic cyclic conditions at a functionally relevant frequency, i.e. in the range of 0.5-3 Hz. The value of the dynamic shear modulus $|G^*|$ for human articular cartilage was found to increase with cyclic frequency, and for a frequency range of 0.01-20 Hz, it varied from ~0.1 to 2.5 MPa (Mankin et al. 1994). In contrast, when cartilage was placed under a constant compressive load for a few hours (i.e. with the interstitial fluid allowed to escape freely), the swelling pressure vanished and the quasi-static compressive modulus was determined to be ~0.4-1.5 MPa (Mankin et al. 1994).

Determining cartilage mechanical properties by indentation testing.

Well-established indentation testing procedures are available for estimating of mechanical properties, typically stiffness and strength. These tests were originally developed in the material sciences for both hard solids (e.g., ceramics and metals) with more recent application to polymeric materials and are increasingly being applied to studies of biologic tissues. Clinical indentation testing devices used for evaluating the mechanical properties of articular cartilage typically employ flat-end cylindrical or spherical probes of a few millimeters in diameter (Appleyard et al. 2001; Aspden et al. 1991; Lyyra et al. 1999; Shepherd and Seedhom 1997; Tkaczuk 1986). Such large-scale clinical indenters average the mechanical properties of the biological tissue over a large volume (mm^3) of material. Hence the sensitivity of resolving local variations in cartilage properties is quite limited, such that, for example, no statistically significant difference was found between clinically healthy and unhealthy types of arthritic cartilage (Tkaczuk 1986).

As the lateral size of the indentation probe decreases, lower forces and penetration depths can often be used, resulting in the measurement of biomechanical properties of a smaller volume of material, potentially with improved sensitivity to local property variations. Thus, when articular cartilage tissue is tested mechanically at the millimeter and micrometer scales, the nanoscale structural components share the task of load bearing, resulting in aggregate mechanical properties that are distinctly different from those of the individual nanoscale components. In contrast, a nanometer-sized AFM tip, being smaller than the diameter of a collagen fiber, can be expected to reveal stiffness variations that are related to the 3-dimensional organization of collagen fibers and proteoglycan chains. Therefore, the combination of micrometer-sized and nanometer-sized AFM tips can be used to measure the aggregate stiffness of articular cartilage as well as the stiffness related to the tissue's fine structure.

Other considerations in tissue indentation testing.

The onset of tip-sample contact in indentation testing is difficult to detect for soft biological tissues, because, compared to hard materials, biological materials are four to six orders of magnitude lower in stiffness and can have more irregular surfaces. These characteristics result in load-displacement data with no abrupt increase in load to mark the point of physical contact. This difficulty was overcome by calculating the area under the load-displacement curves that corresponds to the work done by the cantilever (A-Hassan et al. 1998). Using this approach, a method was established for relative microelastic mapping of living cells.

Because tissues are highly anisotropic and inhomogeneous and thus exhibit site- and direction-specific mechanical properties single-location measurements may yield a significantly biased view of the mechanical properties of a given tissue. Thus, quantitative estimation of any mechanical property is best based on statistical analysis of many repeated measurements. Nevertheless, most published indentation measurements to date of the elastic properties of tissue have been based on the manual selection of one or only a few load-displacement curves. For example, Weisenhorn (Weisenhorn et al. 1993b) employed this approach in IT AFM measurements to determine the elastic modulus of cells and cartilage. Radmacher (Radmacher 1997; Randall et al. 1998) and A-Hassan (A-Hassan et al. 1998) provided information about the contribution of the cytoskeleton to the local cell stiffness of living cells by recording single load-displacement curves at only a few different cell surface locations. Some investigations have also evaluated the effect of drugs on the local stiffness of living cells in this manner (Hoh and Schoenenberger 1994; Rotsch and Radmacher 2000).

Vanlandingham (VanLandingham et al. 1999; VanLandingham et al. 1997a) used the AFM for characterizing the nm-scale properties of the interphase regions of fiber-reinforced polymers. These authors clearly stated that in these systems the nm-scale properties can be significantly different from the bulk properties of one and the same sample. Along the same lines, Rho and Turner (Rho et al. 1997; Turner et al. 1999) measured the elastic properties of human cortical and trabecular lamella bone by nanoindentation using tissue sections dehydrated in a graded series of alcohol solutions. They proposed that the elastic properties of the microstructural components of bone might not be the same as the corresponding macroscopic values. Moreover, they stated that a technique by which elastic properties of the individual microstructural components can be measured would be of great value in understanding the microstructural mechanical behavior of bone. A further step in this direction was made by Hengsberger (Hengsberger et al. 2002) who applied a combination of AFM and a commercial nano-indenter device to measure the influence of the lamella type on the mechanical behavior of cortical and trabecular bone. These measurements, which were performed both under dry and more physiological conditions, revealed a clear dependence on lamella thickness, with thin and thick lamella exhibiting a different mechanical behavior.

The potential for elucidating the changes in structure-mechanical property relationships of cartilage from the millimeter to the micrometer to the nanometer scale motivated us to develop and scrutinize an AFM-based approach (Stolz et al. 1999) to image cartilage and measure its stiffness. We refer to our method as indentation-type AFM (IT AFM). More specifically, we have established and used a protocol for absolute measurements of $|E^*|$, the dynamic elastic modulus, of articular cartilage at two different length scales of tissue organization – micrometer and nanometer – and related our findings to those reported at the millimeter scale.

5.5 Materials and methods

Chemicals.

Unless specified otherwise, all chemicals used were of analytical or best grade available and purchased from one source (Fluka Chemie, Buchs, Switzerland). For all experiments ultrapure deionized water was used (18 MΩ/cm, Brandstead, Boston, USA).

Agarose gel preparation.

Gels were prepared with 0.75%, 2.0%, 2.5% and 3.0% (w/w) agarose (AGAR Noble, DIFCO Laboratories, Detroit MI, USA) in water. For testing agarose gels using IT AFM, plastic rings used to reinforce paper punch holes (inner ring diameter ~5 mm; outer ring diameter ~12 mm; thickness ~0.08 mm) were glued onto 10 mm diameter stainless steel disks used as specimen supports for mounting samples magnetically in the AFM. An aliquot of melted agarose was then poured into the center of the plastic ring and allowed to spread and solidify. The agarose gel was covered with a droplet of water to avoid dehydration. For macro-scale calibration studies described later, gels were poured into cylindrical wells (43 mm diameter x 82 mm height) The hardened gels were removed from the wells immediately before measuring their stiffness.

Cartilage sample preparation.

Porcine articular cartilage was obtained from freshly slaughtered pigs and kept on ice until use. It was prepared from disarticulated knee joints within 1-2 hours post mortem.

The cartilage was harvested from the medial and lateral femoral knee condyles by cutting samples off the underlying bone with a sharp razor blade, yielding ~5 mm x 5 mm pieces that were ~2 mm in thickness. The specimens, usually harvested from several animals at once, were stored at room temperature in PBS (2.6 mM NaH_2PO_4, 3 mM Na_2HPO_4, 155 mM NaCl, 0.01% NaN_3 w/v, pH 7.0) supplemented with a protease inhibitor cocktail (Complete, Boehringer Mannheim, Germany).

Fresh cartilage samples were embedded in Tissue-Tek (Tissue-Tek, 4583 Compound, Sakura Finetek Europe, Zoeterwoude, Netherlands) and sectioned with a cryostatic microtome (SLEE, Mainz, Germany) at -15 °C. From the ~5 mm x 5 mm pieces, ~2 mm in thickness, the outermost (~1 mm thick) layer of the cartilage surface was discarded to minimize surface irregularities and tilt. Then, 20 µm thick frozen sections were allowed to adhere to glass cover slips (6 mm diameter) that had been coated with a 0.01% Poly-L-Lysine solution (Sigma, P 8920) and dried in an oven at 60°C. After adherence, the sections were dried on a hotplate at 40°C.

In preparing cartilage samples for stiffness measurements a Teflon® disk (11 mm diameter x 0.25 mm thick) was first fixed onto a 10 mm diameter stainless steel disk with fast-setting glue (Loctite 401, Henkel KG, Düsseldorf, Germany). Subsequently, the pieces of cartilage described above (~5 mm x 5 mm x 2 mm) were glued onto the Teflon disc with Histoacryl® tissue glue (B. Braun Surgical GmbH, 34209 Melsungen, Germany). The mounted specimens were then placed in a vibratory microtome (752 M Vibroslice, Campden Instruments, Loughborough, UK) to trim off the outermost, ~1 mm thick cartilage layer parallel to the support surface. These trimmed cartilage samples were kept in PBS at 4°C until further use.

Enzymatic digestion of articular cartilage.

For enzymatic digestion of the proteoglycan moiety, a 10 µl droplet of cathepsin D solution (10 U/100 µl diluted in water; Sigma C3138) was applied to a mounted cartilage sample that had been prepared for stiffness measurements and covered with 50 µl of PBS to prevent drying. Similarly, for enzymatic digestion of the collagen fibers, a 10 µl droplet of elastase solution (Leukocyte; 1 U/100 µl diluted in water; Sigma E8140) was applied to a mounted cartilage sample that has been prepared for stiffness measurements and covered with 50 µl of PBS to prevent drying. The specimen was then placed in a Petri dish at saturated humidity and incubated for ~24 hours at 37°C. Three samples were treated and measured independently. Also, three independent controls without enzyme were prepared in parallel. After 24 hours, the enzyme solution was replaced by a drop of PBS. Prior to stiffness measurements, samples were left to equilibrate in PBS for at least 30 min in the fluid cell of the AFM. After completion of the AFM measurement, the 50 μl aliquot of the originally used buffer-enzyme solution was added back to the sample for another ~24 hour incubation prior to a second AFM measurement.

Atomic force microscopy imaging and indentation.

All AFM experiments were carried out with a Nanoscope III (Veeco, Santa Barbara, CA, USA) equipped with a 120-μm scanner (J-scanner) and a standard fluid cell. Images of articular cartilage topography were obtained in AFM contact mode at a scanning rate of ~2 Hz, either in air on dehydrated thin-sectioned samples or in the same PBS buffer solution used for the stiffness measurements but prior to indentation testing. For nanometer scale experiments, oxide sharpened square-based pyramidal silicon nitride tips with a nominal tip radius ~20 nm on V-shaped 200 μm long silicon nitride cantilevers with a nominal spring constant of 0.06 N/m (Veeco) were employed. For micrometer-scale experiments, spherical tips were prepared by gluing borosilicate glass spheres (radius = 2.5 μm; SPI Supplies, West Chester, PA, USA) with epoxy resin (Epicote 1004, Shell Chemicals Ltd, London, UK) onto the end of V-shaped tipless silicon nitride cantilevers having nominal spring constants of 0.06 N/m (Veeco) or 13 N/m (Ultralevers, ThermoMicroscopes, Sunnyvale CA, USA), using a three-dimensional microtranslation stage as described in more detail by Raiteri (Raiteri et al. 1998).

AFM stiffness measurements were based on recording the elastic response of the material by using the AFM tip as either a micro or nano-indenter, depending on which tips were used. Cyclic load-displacement curves (Cappella et al. 1997; Weisenhorn et al. 1993a; Weisenhorn et al. 1992) were recorded at different sites on the sample surface at a vertical displacement frequency of 3 Hz. In order to achieve a constant and well-defined maximum applied load, a maximum tip deflection value (in units of photodiode voltage) was set, where this value (the so-called trigger voltage) indicates the desired increase in photodiode voltage beyond that for the undeflected cantilever probe. In order get the deflection value in nanometers, the optical lever system had to be calibrated for a given tip. For this calibration, load-displacement curves were recorded with the same cantilever on a mica surface, which acted as an "infinitely stiff" sample, i.e., a sample that the tip of a low-stiffness cantilever probe cannot penetrate or deform in any way. The resulting slope obtained for the region of linear compliance provided the "sensitivity" factor, i.e. the factor relating photodiode voltage to nanometers of displacement, for the optical lever system (Cleveland et al.; Gibson et al.; Torii et al.). This "sensitivity" value was used to correct the load-displacement data to obtain load-indentation data (Weisenhorn et al. 1993b).

The load-displacement curves were recorded at different trigger deflections for the two types of indenter tips: at 30 nm for the sharp pyramidal tips, and at 250 nm for the microspherical tips. A trigger deflection of 30 nm with the sharp tips corresponded to an applied load of ~1.8 nN (with k = 0.06 N/m) and maximum penetration depth of, for example, ~550 nm in 0.75% agarose gel and ~300 nm in articular cartilage. A trigger deflection of 250 nm with the spherical tips corresponded to an applied load of ~15 nN (with k = 0.06 N/m) or ~3.3 µN (with k = 13 N/m) and maximum penetration depth of, for example, ~250 nm in 2.5% agarose gel or ~600 nm in cartilage. In all cases, the penetration depths were less than 1% of the sample thickness and thus well below Bueckle's indentation depth limit (10% of specimen thickness) (Bueckle 1973; Persch et al. 1994).

Data acquisition and processing.

The AFM was operated in the so-called "Force-Volume Mode" for recording a set of loading/ unloading load-displacement curves dynamically at a frequency of 3 Hz. In these measurements, an individual set of data consisted of 1,024 load-displacement curves recorded at a given sample site. Each curve consists of 256 data points. To exclude any possible contribution from plastic (i.e. permanent) deformation, only data from the unloading curves were employed.

Software was developed to estimate a linear slope for each curve by fitting a 90°-angle triangle to the unloading part of the load-displacement curve and using its hypotenuse (i.e. the slope of the unloading curve) as a measure of stiffness, S (see dashed line in Fig. 1). The calculated slopes from a given set of 1,024 measurements were plotted as a histogram to which a Gaussian curve was fit (see Fig. 7A). The maximum of the Gaussian curve represents the most frequent S, i.e. S_{max}. Curves within a surrounding interval of $S_{max} \pm 1\%$ (typically 100-200 load-displacement curves) were selected and arithmetically averaged to yield $\bar{S}$.

Determining stiffness using microspherical tips.

For data collected with the microspherical tips, the dynamic elastic modulus $|E^*|$ was computed from the average slope $\bar{S}$ (see Fig. 1) from a set of cyclic load-displacement curves according to the modeling method developed by Oliver and Pharr (Oliver and Pharr

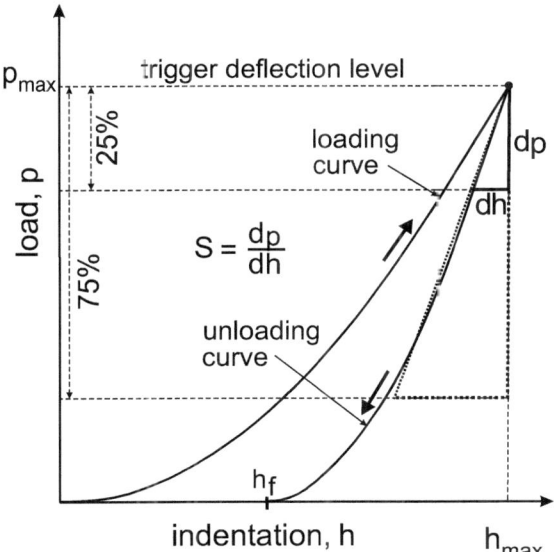

FIGURE 1: Schematic representation of a load-indentation curve during the first complete cycle of loading and unloading. p_{max} is the maximum applied load, p, at maximal indentation depth, h_{max}, and S = dh/dp is the slope of the hypotenuse. In ITAFM measurements of cartilage the slope of the upper 75% of the unloading curve (dashed line) was used for the analysis of the unloading data recorded by employing a sharp pyramidal tip. When employing a micrometer-sized spherical indenter, S was the slope of the upper 25% of the unloading curve (bold line).

1992). In this approach, the upper part of the unloading data can be fitted using a simple power-law equation

$$p = B \cdot (h - h_f)^m$$

where p is the indenter load, h is the vertical displacement of the indenter, and h_f represents the final unloading depth, although it is typically used as a fitting parameter along with B and m (Oliver and Pharr 1992; Sneddon 1965). For spherical indenters, m = 1.5, and for pyramidal tip geometries, m = 2 (VanLandingham et al. 1997a; VanLandingham et al. 1997b).

The load was obtained by simple multiplication of the cantilever deflection with the spring constant k. Next, a power law fit to the average load-indentation curve was determined using the Levenberg-Marquardt algorithm and the stiffness was calculated by linear regression of the upper 25% of this fit. For calculating the dynamic elastic modulus |E*|, we assumed that, |E*| ≈ E where the indentation modulus, E, is given by:

$$E = \frac{\sqrt{\pi}}{2}(1-v^2)\frac{S}{\sqrt{A}}$$

where v is the Poisson's ratio, S the contact stiffness, and A an area function related to the effective cross-sectional or projecting area of the indenter. The Poisson's ratio for agarose gels is $v = 0.5$ (Mak et al. 1987; Matzelle et al. 2002; Vawter). The contact stiffness S = dp/dh has the dimension of force per unit length and is calculated as the derivative of the upper 25% of the unloading part of the load-indentation curve (see Fig. 1).

Determining stiffness using nanometer-scale sharp pyramidal tips.

No attempt was made to model the pyramidal tip data, but rather the slope of the unloading part of the IT AFM load-displacement curve was directly converted into a dynamic elastic modulus by means of a calibration curve recorded from agarose gels. To generate this calibration curve, macro scale measurements of agarose gel stiffness were performed in unconfined compression by following a standard protocol for polymer testing, using a universal mechanical testing apparatus (Zwick Z010; Zwick GmbH, Ulm, Germany). As shown in Fig. 2A, agarose gels exhibit a virtually linear stress-strain behavior over a wide range of applied load. By varying the amount of agarose in the gel (see above) the modulus can be adjusted so as to match the biological tissue of interest (Fig. 2B). Based on the results displayed in Fig. 2, a calibration curve was generated as depicted in Fig. 2C that was used to directly determine the dynamic elastic modulus at the nanometer scale based on the averaged load-displacement curve measured by IT AFM.

5.6 Results

Agarose stiffness was equivalent at both the micrometer and nanometer scale.

Modulus was determined from indentation testing of agarose gels at the nanometer scale with sharp pyramidal tips (radius ~20 nm) based on the calibration curve (Fig. 2C), while modulus determined at the micrometer scale with spherical tips (radius = 2.5 µm) was computed from the load-indentation geometry, as described previously. For a 2.5% agarose gel, the maximum penetration depth reached for the sharp pyramidal tip was ~300 nm and

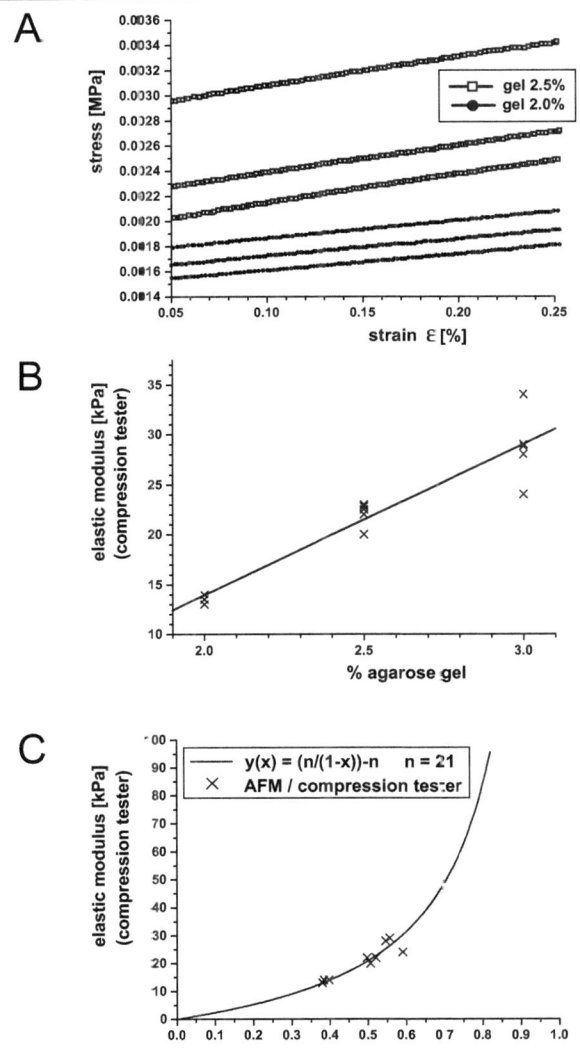

FIGURE 2: Plots of representative data used to develop a calibration curve for the direct conversion of IT AFM load-displacement curves into modulus values; (A) stress-strain data for two agarose gels (2.0% - 3 lower data sets and 2.5% - 3 upper data sets) in compression; (B) modulus values for three agarose gels (2.0%, 2.5%, and 3.0%) measured by compression testing, showing a linear trend with respect to the percent agarose in the gels; (C) the final calibration curve relating the slope of IT AFM load-displacement curves to a corresponding elastic modulus for the three agarose gels (2.0%, 2.5%, and 3.0%). The simplest functional relationship was $y(x) = (n/(1-x))-n$, where $n = 21$ is the fitting parameter, as indicated by the solid curve. A gel with a modulus approaching zero will not bend the cantilever, so the calibration curve must go through the origin, and for an "infinitely" hard sample, the slope is one; thus the asymptotic behavior.

for the microsphere, it was ~250 nm. The resulting values of dynamic elastic modulus were of 0.022 MPa and 0.036 MPa, respectively. The accuracy of these modulus determinations depends on the accuracy of the values of the cantilever spring constant and the sphere size used in the calculations. According to the supplier, the cantilever spring constants have an uncertainty of up to 50%, even for cantilevers on the same wafer, and the sphere size measurements are only accurate within about 5%. Hence the agarose gel moduli determined at the nanometer and micrometer scale were indistinguishable within the range of error.

Cartilage stiffness was about 100-fold lower at the nanometer scale than at the micrometer scale.

In Fig. 3, load-displacement curves are shown for articular cartilage indented with a sharp AFM tip with a nominal tip-radius ~20 nm (Fig. 3A) and with a spherical tip (radius = 2.5 µm) glued to an AFM cantilever (Fig. 3B). The indentation depths were ~300 nm for the sharp pyramidal tip and ~600 nm for the microsphere, and the resulting modulus values were 0.021 MPa and 2.6 MPa, respectively. For comparison to the values obtained by the calibration curve, the averaged unloading load-indentation curve for the sharp pyramidal tip was also modeled according to the Oliver and Pharr model and a dynamic elastic modulus of 0.027 MPa was calculated for articular cartilage (see Table 2 and Fig. 3A). With the uncertainty of the spring constant mentioned above this calculated value of 0.027 MPa is in good agreement to the 0.021 MPa obtained by the calibration curve. The micrometer scale value of 2.6 MPa is comparable to literature values corresponding to millimeter-scale measurements (Shepherd and Seedhom 1997; Swanepoel et al. 1994; Aspden et al. 1991; Popko et al. 1986; Hori and Mockros 1976), but is two orders of magnitude larger than the nanometer-scale value of 0.021 MPa.

Comparison of the structure of agarose gels and articular cartilage.

In Fig. 4, AFM images recorded with a sharp pyramidal tip are shown for a 2.5% agarose gel (Fig. 4A) and articular cartilage (Fig. 4B). The agarose gel image exhibits almost no structural details. In contrast, the surface of the articular cartilage is highly structured with the collagen fibers being randomly oriented. The 67-nm axial repeat of individual collagen fibers is clearly resolved. In Fig. 5, AFM height (Fig. 5A) and deflection (Fig. 5B) images of native articular cartilage imaged with a microspherical tip are shown. The color-grated scale bar displayed in Fig. 5A represents a height range of 10 µm between black and white. In contrast to Fig. 4B, the microspherical tip was not capable of resolving individual fibers, causing the surface to appear relatively homogenous. The dimensions suggest that the

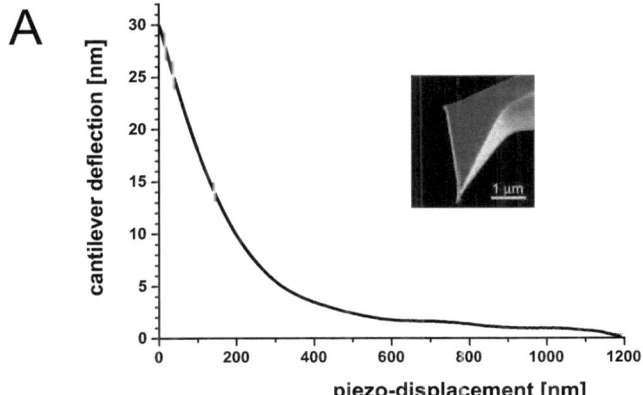

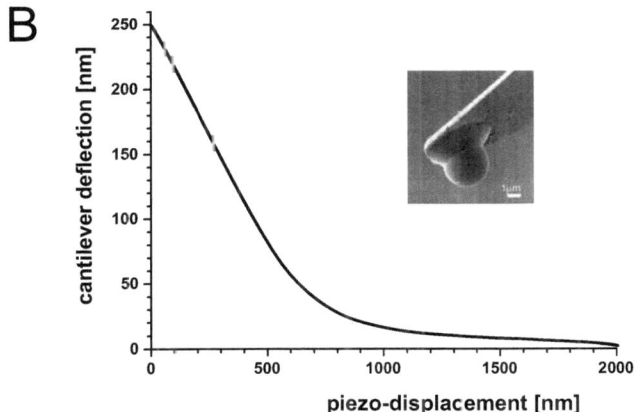

FIGURE 3: Load-displacement curves of articular cartilage recorded with (A) a sharp AFM tip with a nominal tip-radius ~20 nm and (B) a spherical tip glued to an AFM-cantilever (radius = 2.5 µm). Load-displacement curves shown are each based on 1,024 measurements taken at a single site.

structures visible are chondrocytes. Note that imaging of articular cartilage tissue was much more reproducible compared to imaging the agarose gels.

Enzymatic digestion of articular cartilage.

Additional indentation tests were performed at the nanometer and micrometer scales on native articular cartilage to study the effects of the enzymes cathepsin D and elastase. The results are summarized in Table 2. The same protocol as discussed with Fig. 3 was followed, but additionally the articular cartilage was treated with the enzyme cathepsin D for 2 days. As shown in Fig. 6A, no change in stiffness was measured as a result of cathepsin D treatment when employing the microspherical indenter. In contrast, measurements at the nanometer scale revealed stiffening from 0.021 MPa (before treatment) to 0.032 MPa after 1 day, and to 0.054 MPa after 2 days for the same samples (Fig. 6B). In contrast, elastase digestion of collagen significantly reduced the stiffness of cartilage measured at the micrometer scale (Fig. 6C). Articular cartilage samples treated with elastase exhibited a decrease in stiffness from 2.6 MPa (before treatment) to 0.877 MPa after 2 days of exposure. Measurements at the nanometer scale of elastase treated articular cartilage were not possible, because the sample became sticky so that tip-sample adhesion dominated the load-displacement data.

Assessment of IT AFM stiffness measurements.

To assess the sensitivity and reproducibility of stiffness measurements made using IT AFM, large numbers of load-displacement curves were made on three different materials, mica, agarose gels and cartilage. Mica, a stiff, structurally simple material, is an aluminosilicate mineral that is readily cleaved into thin sheets with almost atomically smooth surfaces having little in-plane structural variation above the atomic crystalline level over relatively large areas (millimeter scale or greater). Although mica is softer than many minerals, its stiffness is orders of magnitude higher than the IT AFM cantilever spring constant of $k = 0.06$ N/m, and therefore essentially no penetration of the indenter into the surface occurs. Agarose gels, representing a soft, simple material, have little structure above the atomic scale but are orders of magnitude softer than mica. Cartilage, representing a soft, structurally complex material, is similar in stiffness to agarose gel but exhibits a well-known complex, hierarchical structure, starting at the molecular level and culminating in matrix-embedded fibers visible at low optical magnifications.

A set of 1,024 load-displacement curves were recorded at a single site and the slopes put into a histogram for each of these materials, as shown in Fig. 7A. The width of the Gaussian distributions of calculated slopes was smallest for mica, larger for the agarose gel and largest

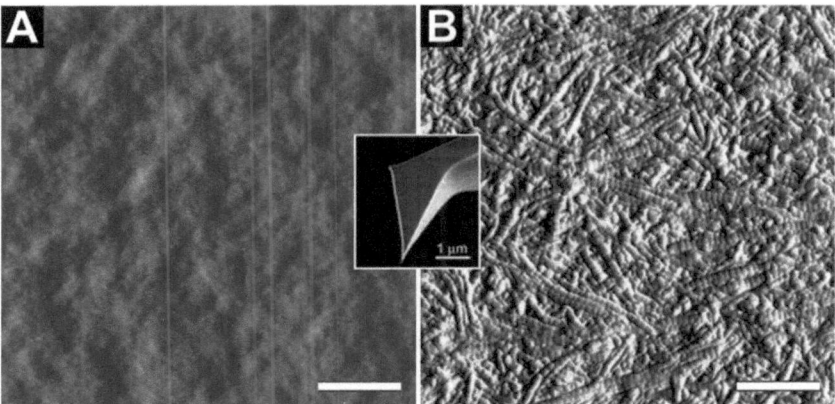

FIGURE 4: Comparison of the structure of (A) an agarose gel (2.5% agarose) with that of (B) articular cartilage as imaged using a sharp AFM tip with a nominal tip radius of ~20 nm. The images demonstrate what the indentation tip "sees" at the nanometer scale. (A) The agarose gel was imaged under aqueous solution, while the articular cartilage was imaged both under buffer solution and after cryo-thin-sectioning in air. Because of the higher resolution the image in air is presented here. The scale bars represent a distance of 1 µm.

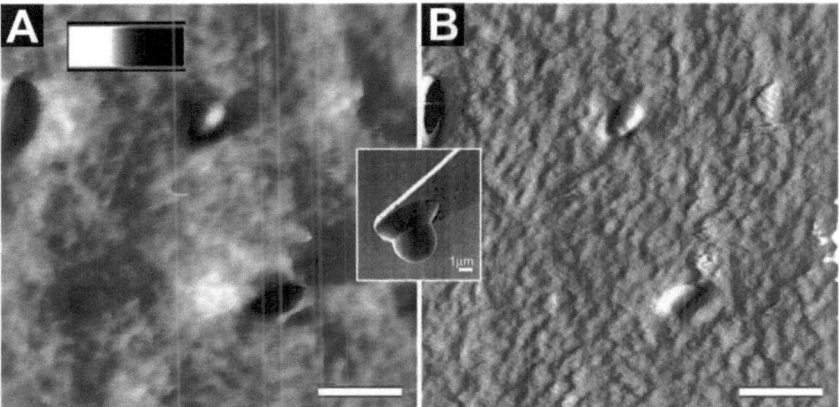

FIGURE 5: AFM images of native articular cartilage imaged in buffer using the microspherical tip: (A) topographic or height image and (B) deflection image. The height range (bar from white to black in (A)) is 10 µm and the scale bars represent a distance of 20 µm.

for the articular cartilage tissue. The corresponding histograms for the digested articular cartilage (i.e. with cathepsin D or elastase; see above) typically were even wider (not shown) than that for the native cartilage. In Fig. 7B, the unloading part of the averaged load-displacement curves is shown as calculated from the curves within a surrounding interval of S_{max} ±1% from each of the histograms in Fig. 7A. The averaged load-displacement curve as shown in Fig. 7B obtained on the hard mica surface exhibits a clear point of tip-sample contact, i.e. a sharp transition between the data prior to contact and after contact. In contrast, the transitions of the averaged unloading load-displacement curves of the agarose gel and cartilage do not exhibit a clear point of contact. The three different unloading load-displacement curves also demonstrate the wide range of indentation depths (i.e. the piezo displacements in Fig. 7B) that may be obtained for the same maximum load (i.e. the maximal cantilever deflection in Fig. 7B) for materials having different stiffnesses.

In addition to single measurements on different materials, IT AFM measurements were made to compare single site measurements to multiple site measurements on cartilage. First, 1,024 unloading load-displacement curves were recorded at a single site of the cartilage tissue; the resulting histogram is shown in Fig. 8A. Then, the AFM scan size was changed from 0x0 µm (collection of unloading load-displacement curves at a single site) to 5x5 µm (collection of 1024 unloading load-displacement curves in a 2-dimensional regular array, i.e. at 156 nm spatial intervals in x and y). More specifically, the AFM tip was advanced to its new position after each loading/ unloading cycle so that 32 lines of 32 unloading load-displacement curves per line were recorded for a total of 1,024 multiple-site curves; the resulting histogram is shown in Fig. 8B. Comparing these two histograms, the width is much larger for the multiple site histogram, and the peak of the corresponding Gaussian distribution curve occurred at a slightly higher modulus value compared to the single site distribution curve although the difference in mean values was not statistically significant. The stiffness distribution for cartilage is also wider than for agarose gels (data not shown), reflecting the less-uniform structure of cartilage. Additionally, kinks were often observed in the load-displacement curves for cartilage apparently due to changes in the local deformation process related to the heterogeneous structure. Repeated multiple site measurements at a scan size 5x5 µm revealed that the most frequent modulus and the shape of the Gaussian distribution were highly reproducible (data not shown).

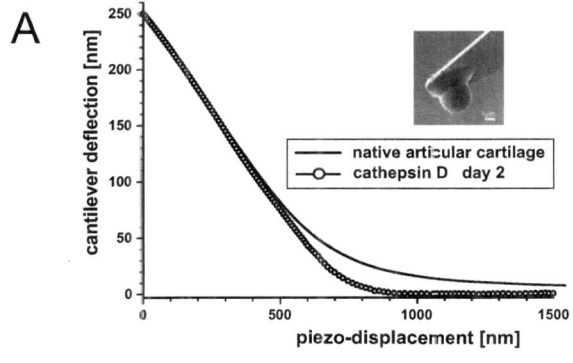

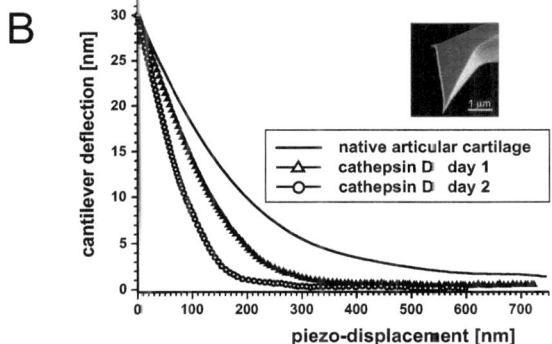

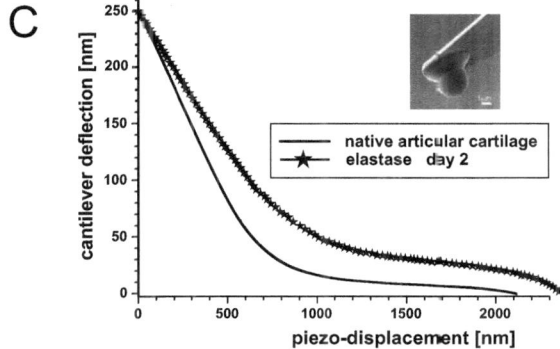

FIGURE 6: Load-displacement curves comparing the response of articular cartilage before and after enzymatic digestion with cathepsin D (A and B) and elastase (C). In (A) and (C), measurements were made using the microsphere tip, while in (B) measurements were made using sharp pyramidal tip. The same samples (n = 3) were evaluated using both indenter sizes; however, measurements on elastase digested cartilage using the sharp pyramidal tip was not feasible, due to the tip sticking in the digested cartilage.

5.7 Discussion

Indentation testing of soft biological materials.

This study represents the first exploratory investigation of dimensional scale on the measured stiffness of soft biological tissues by IT AFM. Our goal was to make indentation testing of soft biological tissues both more reproducible and also capable of evaluating the effects of changes in fine structure on tissue stiffness – both mean values and site-to-site variability. These considerations resulted in a new protocol for preparing and mechanically testing articular cartilage in a mode that maintains its *bona fide* structure and its biological functioning. Because articular cartilage is a load bearing tissue, our protocol for measuring its dynamic elastic modulus including physiologically relevant loading rates.

In order to extract meaningful indentation data for soft biological specimens, a variety of difficulties related to the special nature of these materials, including differences to indentation testing of hard solids, needed to be considered. First, some traditional indentation testing protocols include the use of preloads prior to loading and/ or long hold periods prior to unloading to reduce time-dependent effects on the resulting data. However, preloading of soft biological tissue would inevitably move the water within the tissue. Also, because articular cartilage is a highly viscoelastic material, its functional stiffness, the dynamic elastic modulus $|E^*|$, is most appropriately determined from either stress relaxation as a function of time or cyclic load-displacement data as a function of frequency. For providing stiffness data relevant to the function of the knee joint, the cyclic rate employed should reflect the transient loading/ unloading time of normal ambulation (walking, running). For articular cartilage this is in the range of a few hundred milliseconds (Popko et al. 1986; Shepherd and Seedhom 1997). Therefore, we performed indentation testing at 3 Hz (three complete loading/ unloading cycles per second), corresponding to an indenter unloading time of about 150 milliseconds.

Oliver and Pharr have demonstrated that the elastic modulus of solid materials can be derived by modeling load-indentation curves as illustrated in Fig. 1 within a few percent (Oliver and Pharr 1992; Pharr and Oliver 1992; Pharr et al. 1992). In determination of the elastic modulus of hard solid materials, indentation depths are extremely low and consequently sharp tips are mostly preferred to other geometries in order to that measurable indentation occurs. However, from our experience a spherical tip shape produces results which are more consistent and easier to model and interpret in testing soft biological specimens. Unfortunately, there are no well-defined spherical indenters available for indentation tests at the sub-cellular level.

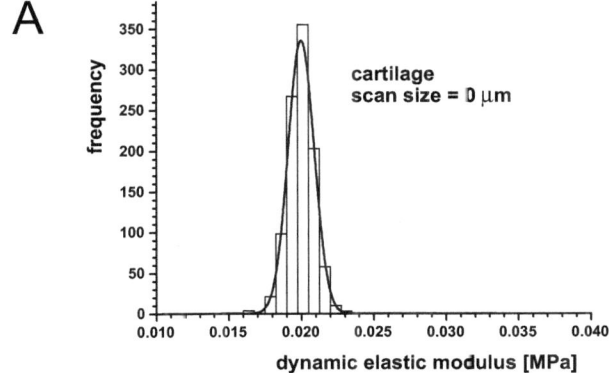

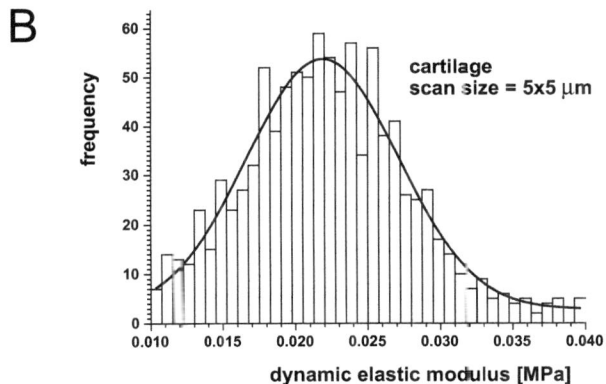

FIGURE 7: (A) Histograms and corresponding Gaussian distribution curves for repeated stiffness measurements on mica, agarose gel, and articular cartilage. Each histogram was based on 1,024 load-displacement curves and was taken at a single site. (B) Averaged unloading load-displacement curves for the three different materials corresponding to the curves within ± 1% of the frequency peak in (A).

To date, stiffness measurements by AFM on biological samples have been most commonly interpreted based on the Hertz model (A-Hassan et al. 1998; Radmacher 1997; Radmacher et al. 1995; Rotsch et al. 1999; Vinckier and Semenza 1998; Walch et al. 2000). While the Hertz model analyzes the problem of the elastic contact between two spherical surfaces

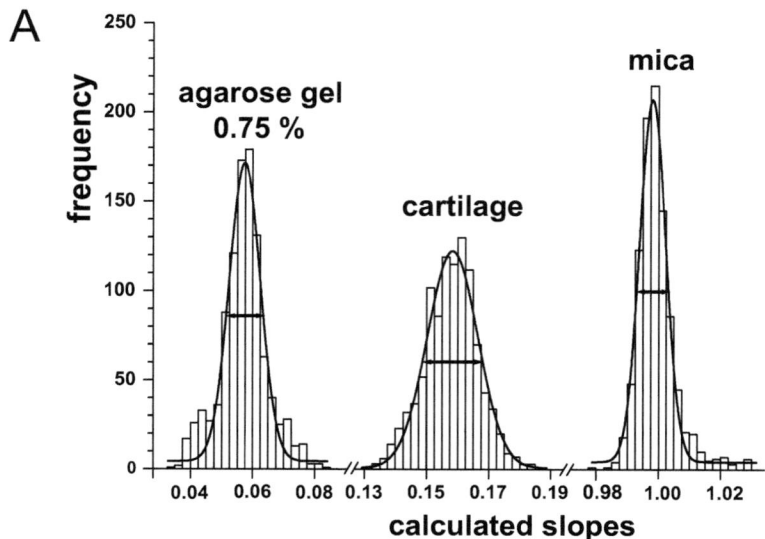
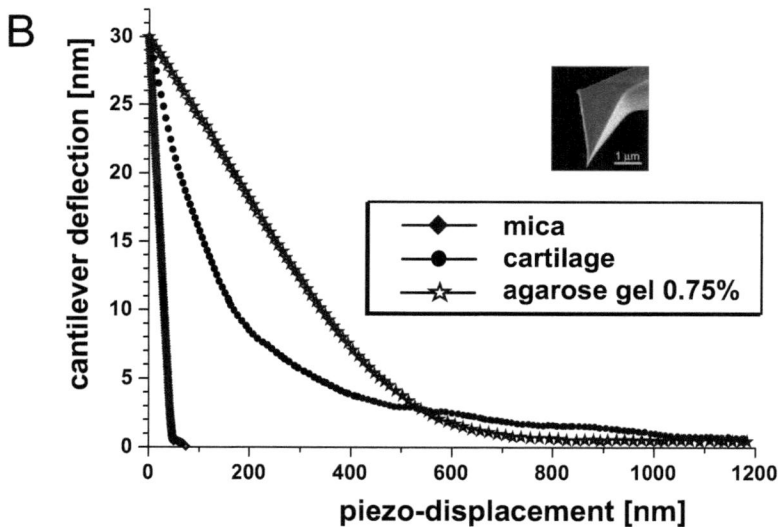

FIGURE 8: Histograms and corresponding Gaussian distribution curves for (A) 1,024 stiffness measurements at a single site, i.e. at scan size 0, and (B) 1,024 stiffness measurements at multiple sites spaced evenly over a 5x5 μm area. The data were taken at the nanometer scale on porcine articular cartilage.

with different radii and elastic constants (Hertz 1882; Sneddon 1965), most AFM-based indentation experiments have been performed with sharp pyramidal tips (radius ~5-30 nm). Further, inherent in these analyses is the need to precisely locate the initial point of contact between the tip and the specimen surface. However, for soft biological tissues, the accurate determination of the point of contact was recently described to be "one of the most vexing problems" (A-Hassan et al. 1998). Compared to hard materials, soft biological tissues are several orders of magnitude lower in stiffness and can have more irregular surfaces due to the lack of sample preparation, so that there is no abrupt increase in load to mark the point of physical contact. To achieve meaningful data for soft biological tissues, higher depth/ width ratio indents need to be made with sharp pyramidal tips compared to, for example, spherical tips to minimize effects of tip-sample adhesion forces. Unfortunately, sharp tip indentation (tip radius << indentation depth) causes complicated stress-strain fields in the tissue under the tip that is not accounted for by the Hertzian model.

To avoid some of these issues, calibration with reference materials can be used. In fact, calibration procedures for indentation of hard materials typically include indentation of reference samples. While hard materials can be cut and machined to produce specimens suitable for indentation testing at different dimensional scales, biological tissues are limited in their dimensions by anatomic location and function. Therefore, agarose gels can be used as a tissue-like reference material because they (i) represent a high water content organic material, that is readily modeled as a mechanically isotropic structure at the length scales of interest (i.e. at the nanometer and micrometer scale), (ii) can be prepared in a standard and reproducible manner, and (iii) are available in bulk quantities. Further, because the gel properties vary as a function of gel content, a calibration curve can be created such as the local geometry of the tip and the profile of the sample deformation does not need to be known. The disadvantage of a calibration curve is that the sample measurement is only accurate for exactly the same set of parameters, and the same tip with the same cantilever spring constant as were used for determining the calibration curve. Hence, every time a new tip shape, cantilever spring constant, indentation speed or indentation depth is employed, a new calibration curve must be determined.

In IT AFM determination of the elastic properties of biological materials, extraneous phenomena such as adhesion forces between the tip and sample or electrostatic interactions may cause irregularities in the lower part of the load-displacement curve (i.e. at low physical contact of the tip with the surface), thereby adding substantial "noise" to the recorded signal. To derive as much reliable information from the load-displacement curves as possible, the data from the upper 75% (percentage relative to the maximum force) of the unloading curves were used, because they were essentially noise free and appeared reproducible over many indentation and retraction cycles on different biological samples. Also, no post-indentation deformation was evident that could have compromised the upper portion of the unloading curve.

sample	indenter shape radius (nominal values)	spring constant [N/m] (nominal values)	method	(dynamic) elastic modulus ± variation [MPa] / number of measurements (n)	
agarose 2.5 %	flat-punch cylindrical r > 3 cm	–	compression tester	E = 0.022 ± 0.002 / 3	
	spherical r = 2.5 µm	k = 0.06	modeling	$|E^*|$ = 0.036 ± 0.005 / 3	
	pyramidal r = 20 nm	k = 0.06	blind calib	$|E^*|$ = 0.022 ± 0.003 / 5	
articular cartilage (native)	spherical r = 2.5 µm	k = 13	modeling	$|E^*|$ = 2.6 ± 0.05 / 4	
	pyramidal r = 20 nm	k = 0.06	modeling	$|E^*|$ = 0.027 ± 0.003 / 5	
	pyramidal r = 20 nm	k = 0.06	blind calib	$|E^*|$ = 0.021 ± 0.003 / 5	
articular cartilage cat D digestion	spherical r = 2.5 µm	k = 13	modeling	$|E^*|$ = 2.6 ± 0.05 / 4	0#
				$|E^*|$ = 2.6 ± 0.05 / 4	2#
	pyramidal r = 20 nm	k = 0.06	blind calib	$|E^*|$ = 0.021 ± 0.003 / 5	0#
				$|E^*|$ = 0.032 ± 0.006 / 5	1#
				$|E^*|$ = 0.054 ± 0.010 / 5	2#
articular cartilage elastase digestion	spherical r = 2.5 µm	k = 13	modeling	$|E^*|$ = 2.6 ± 0.05 / 4	0#
				$|E^*|$ = 0.877 ± 0.05 / 4	2#
	pyramidal r = 20 nm	k = 0.06	blind calib	(i)	

Elasticity measurements done after 0, 1 or 2 days of cathepsin D or elastase digestion

TABLE 2: Comparison of the dynamic elastic modulus $|E^*|$ of a 2.5% agarose gel and for native, cathepsin D digested and elastase digested articular cartilage. Values are shown for nanometer-sized sharp pyramidal tips and micrometer-sized spherical tips employed for the IT AFM measurements, along with values determined for the agarose gel with a millimeter-sized compression tester. For IT AFM measurements, modulus values were determined from the slopes of the load-displacement curves using either an elasticity-based indentation model (modeling) or a calibration curve based on compression testing of agarose gels (blind calibration). The data on articular cartilage are the result of measurements on articular cartilage that came from pig knees of several different animals. The number of data sets, n, averaged to produce a given tabulated value is shown.

(i) After digestion of the sample with elastase, it became very sticky so that reliable measurements of the modulus were not possible.

Specimen stability and integrity.

A prerequisite to performing IT AFM of soft biological tissues is the stable immobilization of the sample on a solid support in a close-to-native state. Because specimens can easily deteriorate during preparation or inspection, the protocol devised has to maintain the integrity of the biological structure upon immobilization. Immobilization of the specimens on a solid support must be stable, yet the chemistry of the adhesive or glue should not alter the structural and/ or functional properties of the specimen.

For indentation tests using nanometer-sized indenters on hard solids, ultra-smooth surfaces can often be prepared by finely polishing the sample with abrasive compounds of decreasing grain sizes in liquid suspensions. In contrast, for indentation testing of soft biological tissues their natural surfaces are often intrinsically neither smooth nor homogeneous at the nanometer scale. For assessing inner zones of a tissue, the outer layer can be removed by sectioning, but this still does not ensure a smooth surface at this scale. In IT AFM, a rough surface in combination with the low cantilever spring constants required for low-stiffness materials inevitably adds more noise to the measurement. To compensate, much larger indentation depths (producing longer load-displacement curves) were needed for indentation testing the agarose gels or articular cartilage compared to the measurement of hard solids. Moreover, biological specimen surfaces are typically charged. The electrostatic interactions between the surface and the tip and local variations in the ion content of the buffer at the nanometer scale add more noise to the measurement. This is another reason why deeper indents are required.

The use of relatively large penetration depth might have caused fluid flow within or out of the cartilage during the dynamic tests. However, load-displacement curves obtained during unloading and recorded at 3 Hz using either microsphere or the sharp pyramidal tip on both agarose gels and articular cartilage did not change over the course of our multiple cycle protocol. Even after hundreds of loading and unloading cycles, no changes were observed in the load-displacement behavior, nor were any persistent residual indentations (which would be indicative of yield and plastic flow) or any mechanical effects or imaging appearance changes indicative of material fatigue. Given this lack of change in mechanical properties, the hypothesis regarding the absence of fluid flow within or out of the cartilage during the dynamic tests appears sufficiently correct. Also, given the absence of signs of structural damage and the apparently complete dimensional recovery of the samples, the use of elastic contact theory for the data analysis appears to be at least a good first approximation (Oliver and Pharr 1992).

Determining representative load-displacement curves.

The IT AFM stiffness measurements at the nanometer scale were compared for three different materials exhibiting different combinations of hierarchical structural complexity and stiffness – mica, an agarose gel, and articular cartilage. Comparison between the histograms as documented in Fig. 7A of the slopes of individual load-displacement curves of the hard mica, the homogeneous agarose gels and the multiphasic cartilage biocomposite reveals a broadening of the distribution with decreasing stiffness and increasing complexity of the sample. The widths of the Gaussian distributions Fig. 7A also demonstrate the difficulty of selecting a representative load-displacement curve for a given sample. Indentation testing of articular cartilage tissue exhibited a much larger variation in the stiffness values as usually performed by the collection of only a few unloading load-displacement curves for characterizing a homogenous hard solid, such as mica.

The width of the stiffness histogram broadens considerably when the 1,024 load-displacement curves are recorded from multiple sample sites (Fig. 8B) rather than measured at a single sample site (Fig. 8A). This result could indicate either an increase in "noise" or an actual variation in modulus due to the sharp tip encountering slightly different arrangements of the complex cartilage structure. However, a tip with a nominal radius of ~20 nm can in principle be positioned on top of a collagen fiber of 50 nm diameter, in-between two fibers, or the tip might interact in many different ways with the collagen fibers. Because of the variety of difficulties related to indentation testing of soft biological tissues that potentially can lead to large variations of the data, we based our results by IT AFM on a large enough number of unloading load-displacement curves followed by statistical analysis.

Comparison of modulus values at the micrometer and nanometer scales.

Indentation testing of a cultured cell that has a thickness of a few micrometers or the articular cartilage in a human knee joint of about 1-4 mm thickness is often limited by the performance of the instrument. However, IT AFM, which is based on piezoelectric actuators, has far greater dimensional sensitivity compared to conventional clinical indentation testing devices for mechanical testing of small samples (see discussion above). Whatever instrumentation is employed for indentation testing, the rule of Bueckle specifies a maximum indentation depth of 10% of the overall thickness of a sample having the same structure throughout. Otherwise, the results vary with the ratio of depth to thickness. Hence for articular cartilage (~1-4 mm thick), the overall z-range (i.e. 0.1-0.4 mm) that remains for testing a specimen often is close to the resolution capability of clinical indentation testing devices. Moreover, some published data might be biased by the presence or absence of an underlying bone or other substrate of different stiffness.

In contrast to clinical indenters that probe cartilage at the millimeter scale, a sharp AFM tip with a radius typically ~20 nm, which is smaller than an individual collagen fiber having a diameter of about 50 nm, was used. With this nanometer-scale indenter, a dynamic elastic modulus of 0.021 MPa was obtained. This value is ~100-fold lower than reported values obtained with millimeter-sized clinical indenters. For example, Hori measured the short-time elastic modulus for human articular cartilage, including both healthy and diseased samples, to vary over 0.4-3.5 MPa and the short-time bulk elastic modulus over the range 9-170 MPa (Hori and Mockros 1976). Popko reported a dynamic elastic modulus for human knee cartilage of 1.5-9.7 MPa, i.e. with the areas of highest weight bearing being characterized by a higher dynamic elastic modulus (Popko et al. 1986). Aspden measured a strain rate dependency for bovine knee articular cartilage from 0.58 MPa to 1.63 MPa (Aspden et al. 1991), and Swanepoel determined a mean stiffness of healthy human lumbar apophyseal cartilage of 2.8 MPa (Swanepoel et al. 1994). Finally, Shepherd reported values of the compressive elastic modulus of human articular knee cartilage under physiological loading rates between 4.4-27 MPa (Shepherd and Seedhom 1997). Interestingly, using a micrometer-size (2.5 µm radius) spherical tip (see Table 2 and Fig. 3B), a dynamic elastic modulus of 2.6 MPa was obtained, a value in close agreement with clinical indenter measurements.

Employing sharp pyramidal tips similar to those used in our measurements, Weisenhorn performed AFM measurements on bovine articular cartilage of the proximal head of the humerus. By modeling the stress-strain curves, an elastic modulus of 0.16-0.6 MPa was calculated (Weisenhorn et al. 1993b). The difference between these stiffness values and those obtained by clinical indenter measurements was explained as being caused by the inhomogeneity of the elastic response. Because cartilage is not a homogenous material, the macro-scale stiffness represents an average of the elastic response of the various structural elements comprising the tissue, whereas at the nanometer scale, the stiffness of the individual structural elements is measured.

To explore this hypothesis that the ~100-fold modulus difference is due to the measurement of the molecular and supramolecular cartilage components at the nanometer and micrometer scales, respectively, the influence of the tip size on image resolution was explored using agarose gels and articular cartilage. As expected, the agarose gels appear amorphous not only at the micrometer scale but also at the nanometer scale (see Fig. 4A). After all, a 2.5%

agarose gel consists of 97.5% water with the 2.5% supporting gel structure being a relatively simple cross-linked galactose polymer. Hence, the agarose gel exhibits a similar stiffness at both the micrometer and nanometer scales. In contrast, the articular cartilage surface imaged at the nanometer scale appears distinctly structured with individual collagen fibers and even their characteristic 67-nm axial repeat length being resolved (see Fig. 4B). In our attempt of imaging articular cartilage under buffer solution we could also resolve individual collagen fibers in a similar quality as previously obtained by Jurvelin (Jurvelin et al. 1999). However, because of the significant lower resolution obtained under buffer conditions, we only present images in air. In Fig. 4B, the collagen fibers appear relatively loosely packed against each other with a random orientation. However, when articular cartilage is imaged with a micrometer-sized spherical tip, its surface topography appears rather featureless (see Fig. 5) – i.e. similar to an agarose gel – except for some chondrocytes that are just barely resolved. These results appear to support the assertion that the ~100-fold difference in articular cartilage stiffness between measurements at the micrometer or nanometer scale is meaningful and reflects differences in the level of structure that is probed – i.e., the cartilage structural elements acting in concert at the supramolecular level versus distinct entities of the molecular level cartilage structure.

Effects of enzymatic digestion on cartilage stiffness.

As might be expected, the chemical and physical states of the proteoglycan (PG) moiety play an important role in defining cartilage pathology. For example, osteoarthritic cartilage exhibits a distinct loss of the PG content (Maroudas 1976). *Ex vivo*, such changes can be induced in a controlled way by specific enzymatic digestion of some components of the PG moiety. In order to assess the contribution of the PG moiety to the stiffness of articular cartilage, specimens were incubated with cathepsin D (Bader and Kempson 1994) and their stiffness was measured at different time points at both the nanometer and micrometer scale. The stiffness determined at the micrometer scale did not exhibit any significant change even after 40 h of enzyme treatment (see Fig. 6A). This result is consistent with the results obtained by Bader and Kempson (Bader and Kempson 1994), who followed the course of a similar cathepsin D digestion experiment of articular cartilage with a macroscopic indenter. Evidently, digestion of the PGs does not significantly affect the bulk elastic properties of articular cartilage. This suggests that although the PGs are fragmented by the enzyme, the PG remnants still foster the ionic imbalance and charge repulsion phenomena that lead to water retention and the swelling that place in the collagen matrix in tension. This result obviously bears further study. In contrast, when measured at the nanometer scale, the stiffness of articular cartilage gradually increased with progressive cathepsin D digestion (see Fig. 6B). Thus, stiffness measurements with a sharp nanometer-sized pyramidal tip appear to be a sensitive means for assessing the structural degradation of the proteoglycan moiety, which intersperses with the fibrous collagen network (see Table 2).

In a related experiment, articular cartilage was incubated for two days with the enzyme elastase, which specifically digests the collagen fibers. In this case, the dynamic elastic modulus measured at the micrometer scale decreased substantially, i.e. from 2.6 MPa to 0.877 MPa (see Table 2 and Fig. 6C), which can clearly be attributed to the destruction of the collagen fibers. Reproducible measurements at the nanometer scale on elastase digested cartilage were not feasible, because the tip became readily contaminated by the digested products and often stuck to the sample surface.

5.8 Conclusions

We have established a technique, which we refer to as IT AFM, for directly measuring the stiffness of cartilage at length scales of both a few nanometers and several micrometers that span much of the range of the hierarchically organized structure of articular cartilage. This technique should be applicable to other tissues also. The IT AFM dynamic elastic modulus of articular cartilage determined with micrometer-sized spherical tips is in good agreement with values obtained by clinical indenters which typically determine stiffness at the millimeter-scale. In contrast, stiffness values measured with IT AFM using nanometer-sized sharp pyramidal tips were typically 100-fold lower. Comparison of the size of the indenters relative to the structural building blocks of cartilage led to the conclusion that this stiffness difference was due to the two distinct levels of tissue organization at these scales. In contrast, when agarose gels, which are more amorphous and elastically isotropic than cartilage, were measured by the same IT AFM technique, the stiffness was the same at the micrometer and nanometer scales within the range of error.

Articular cartilage is a complex composite material, principally comprised of a collagen fiber network placed under tension by the swelling pressure of the proteoglycan gel interspersed within it. The resulting structure is actually mostly water – i.e. 60-80 wt.%. Consequently, the observed mechanical properties of cartilage depend highly on the dimensional level at which they are investigated. Based on our measurements, we conclude that a 2.5 μm radius spherical tip is still large enough to yield information about the bulk elastic behavior of cartilage. In contrast, nanometer-sized tips enable us to observe mechanical properties and structure at the nanometer-scale. For example, while not detectable at the micrometer or millimeter scale, digestion of the cartilage proteoglycan moiety with the enzyme cathepsin D increased the dynamic elastic modulus significantly when measured with nanometer-sized sharp pyramidal tips. In contrast, digestion of the collagen fiber network by elastase decreased the tissue stiffness drastically at the micrometer scale. (Collagen digestion products blocked attempts to make measurements at the nanometer scale.)

More detailed information about the mechanical properties of articular cartilage, including changes that might be triggered by physical and chemical stimuli, may be of practical importance for a better understanding of both cartilage mechanics and cartilage disease progression. Measurements at the nanometer scale provided by sharp pyramidal tips may open the possibility for either early diagnosis of proteoglycan changes related to the onset of cartilage diseases such as osteoarthritis or the effects of pharmaceutical agents on the tissue. Ultimately, this study may be a step toward developing an arthroscopic IT AFM for direct *in vivo* inspection of the articular cartilage at the nanometer scale in a knee or hip joint in a clinical environment (Hunziker et al. 2002). Finally, IT AFM measurements of the functional stiffness of articular cartilage with micrometer-sized spherical tips may also be of clinical interest. Potentially, this method would allow investigations of joint surfaces such as those in the fingers or ankles, where joint surfaces are small and the cartilage is much thinner, i.e., where current clinical millimeter scale indenters are too big.

5.9 Other potential applications in biology, medicine and bioengineering

5.9.1 Quality control of engineered tissue or biomaterials

The future of tissue engineering holds the promise of custom-made parts, supplied by laboratory construction of tissue cultures, tissue-scaffold hybrids and organ cultures. (Langer and Vacanti 1993). The aim is to regenerate damaged or diseased tissue and new biocompatible implants that can be resorbed by the body after its function is done. However, towards broad implications of the intrinsic mechanical properties of those composite biological specimens have to be better understood at the basis of the structural features with their physical and chemical composition and consequently their functionality.

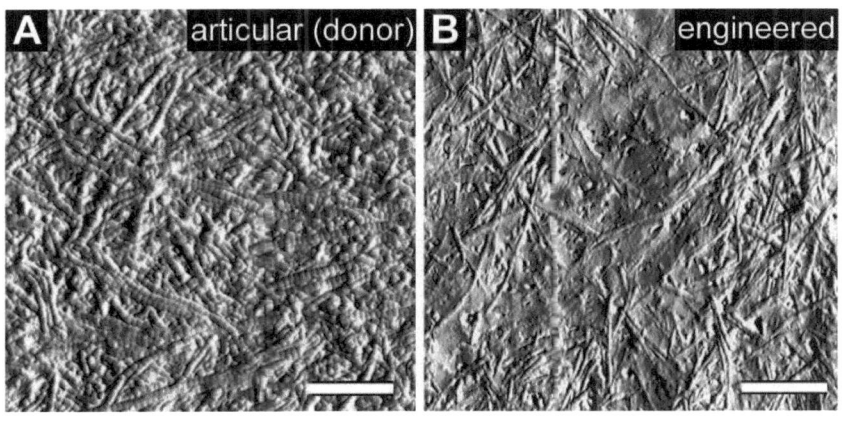

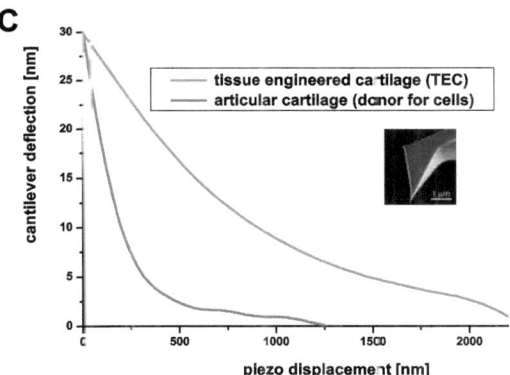

FIGURE 9: Characterization of different types of engineered cartilage for tissue repair or tissue replacement **(A)** AFM image of articular articular cartilage **(B)** AFM image of engineered articular cartilage **(C)** corresponding indentation curves on the engineered articular cartilage (magenta) versus native articular cartilage (green). Scale bar, 1 μm.

In the context of engineered tissue, the use of artificial and bio-like materials, such as implant materials for soft and hard tissue substitution, but also tissue-engineered or heterologous transplants for the replacement of lesions of articular cartilage requires a sensitive, nanoscale to microscale property evaluation. A point of special interest in here is the surface or interface mechanics of soft and hard connective tissues and of engineered biomaterials.

However, an accurate knowledge of the mechanical function of native, stimulated medical repaired or transplanted cartilage tissue or the design, production and long term stability of functional tissue engineered cartilage (TEC) is of major importance. Consequently better analytical tools for appropriate tests and analysis of the biomechanical competence of native, pathological or new synthetic biocompatible materials have to be developed.

As documented in Fig. 9, we employed the AFM as a tool for quality control where the morphology is compared, but also the mechanical properties of authentic articular cartilage with tissue engineered cartilage (TEC) that is produced in a bioreactor, so that it can eventually be used for repair or replacement after trauma or disease. The two curves in Fig. 9B document that the engineered bovine articular cartilage is significant softer (~12 kPa) compared to the native cartilage (~21 kPa) when assayed at the nanometer scale. we started also measurements that assess the biomechanical properties at the micrometer and millimeter scale by employing AFM in combination with compression tester measurements. This part of the work especially addresses the improvement of the biomechanical properties of TEC, so that it becomes better, i.e. in terms of similar properties compared to the native (donor) cartilage.

Moreover, assessing the biomechanical properties of cartilage at the mm, μm and nm scales in combination with biochemical analysis will help us to learn and understand its native properties. This gain in knowledge is a prerequisite for the designing, building and testing an arthroscopic AFM.

5.9.2 Exploring the vulnerability of coronary artery plaques

Another potential application of probing soft biological tissue by IT AFM or by employing multifunctional local probes might be the *in situ* detection and characterization of vulnerable coronary artery plaques, for example, by incorporating AFM-based probes into catheters. Atherosclerosis is a progressing disease that leads to "plaque" formation in arteries supplying critical organs such as the heart or the brain with blood. Two types of plaques exist: (1) vulnerable, lipid-rich plaques prone to mechanical rupture and thus leading to myocardial infarction and stroke; and (2) fibrous, stable plaques rarely being life-threatening (Ross 1986). Conventionally, discrimination of the two types of plaques is done histologically at autopsy (Virmani et al. 2000). In a more futuristic scenario, we might envisage to detect and distinguish these two plaque types *in situ* by catheter-based tools that can probe their distinct mechanical rigidity and local heat production. As with articular cartilage in a first step the elastic properties of such artery plaques have to be assessed *ex vivo* by IT AFM, i.e. by systematically measuring normal, mildly and severely atherosclerotic autopsy specimens. The elastic moduli of these experiments could lead to a reference database being a prerequisite for later *in situ* application of the method using catheter-mounted versions of the multi-functional local probes.

5.5 References

A-Hassan E, Heinz WF, Antonik MD, D'Costa NP, Nageswaran S, Schoenenberger CA, Hoh JH. 1998. Relative microelastic mapping of living cells by atomic force microscopy. *Biophysical Journal* vol.74, no.3; March 1998; p.1564 78.

Appleyard RC, Swain MV, Khanna S, Murrell GA. 2001. The accuracy and reliability of a novel handheld dynamic indentation probe for analysing articular cartilage. *Phys Med Biol* 46(2):541-50.

Armstrong CG, Mow VC. 1982. Variations in the intrinsic mechanical properties of human articular cartilage with age, degeneration, and water content. *J Bone Joint Surg Am* 64(1):88-94.

Aspden RM, Larsson T, Svensson R, Heinegard D. 1991. Computer-controlled mechanical testing machine for small samples of biological viscoelastic materials. *J Biomed Eng* 13(6):521-5.

Bader DL, Kempson GE. 1994. The short-term compressive properties of adult human articular cartilage. *Biomed Mater Eng* 4(3):245-56.

Bueckle H. 1973. The science of hardness testing and its research applications; j.W. Westbrook, h. Conrad (eds.), american society for metals, metals park, ohio.

Cappella B, Baschieri P, Frediani C, Miccoli P, Ascoli C. 1997. Force-distance curves by AFM. A powerful technique for studying surface interactions. *IEEE Eng Med Biol Mag* 16(2):58-65.

Cleveland JP, Manne S, Bocek D, Hansma PK. 1993. A nondestructive method for determining the spring constant of cantilevers for scanning force microscopy. *Review of Scientific Instruments* vol.64(2):p.403 5.

Cohen NP, Foster RJ, Mow VC. 1998. Composition and dynamics of articular cartilage: Structure, function, and maintaining healthy state. *J Orthop Sports Phys Ther* 28(4): 203-15.

Gibson CT, Watson GS, Myhra S. 1996. Determination of the spring constants of probes for force microscopy/ spectroscopy. *Nanotechnology* vol.7, no.3; p.259 62.

Hengsberger S, Kulik A, Zysset P. 2002. Nanoindentation discriminates the elastic properties of individual human bone lamellae under dry and physiological conditions. *Bone* 30(1):178-84.

Hertz H. 1882. Über die berührung fester elastischer körper. *Journal für die reine und angewandte Mathematik* vol. 92, 156–171.

Hoh JH, Schoenenberger CA. 1994. Surface morphology and mechanical properties of MDCK monolayers by atomic force microscopy. *J Cell Sci* 107(Pt 5):1105-14.

Hori RY, Mockros LF. 1976. Indentation tests of human articular cartilage. *J Biomech* 9(4):259-68.

Hues SM, Colton RJ, Meyer E, Guntherodt HJ. 1993. Scanning probe microscopy of thin films. *MRS Bulletin; 18(1): 41 9.*

Hunziker P, Stolz M, Aebi U. 2002. Nanotechnology in medicine: Moving from the bench to the bedside. *Chimia* 56(10):520-526.

Jurvelin JS, Muller DJ, Wong M, Studer D, Engel A, Hunziker EB. 1996. Surface and subsurface morphology of bovine humeral articular cartilage as assessed by atomic force and transmission electron microscopy. *J Struct Biol* 117(1):45-54.

Lai WM, Hou JS, Mow VC. 1991. A triphasic theory for the swelling and deformation behaviors of articular cartilage. *J Biomech Eng* 113(3):245-58.

Langer R, Vacanti JP. 1993. Tissue engineering. *Science* 260(5110):920-6.

Lueke HD. 1992. Modulationsverfahren i, uebertragung digitaler signale; chapter 7 in: Signaluebertragung, grundlagen der digitalen und analogen nachrichtenuebertargungssysteme; 5. Auflage; p. 200 ff; editor: Lueke hd; publisher: Springer verlag Berlin Heidelberg, Germany.

Lyyra T, Arokoski JP, Oksala N, Vihko A, Hyttinen M, Jurvelin JS, Kiviranta I. 1999. Experimental validation of arthroscopic cartilage stiffness measurement using enzymatically degraded cartilage samples. *Phys Med Biol* 44(2):525-35.

Ma PX, Schloo B, Mooney D, Langer R. 1995. Development of biomechanical properties and morphogenesis of in vitro tissue engineered cartilage. *J Biomed Mater Res* 29(12):1587-95.

Mak AF, Lai WM, Mow VC 1987. Biphasic indentation of articular cartilage. I. Theoretical analysis. *Journal of Biomechanics* vol.20; no.7; 1987; p.703 14.

Mankin H, Mow V, Buckwalter J, Iannotti J, Ratcliffe A. 1994. Form and function of articular cartilage; chapter 1 in : Orthopaedic basic science; editor: Simon, sr; publisher: American academy of orthopaedic surgeons; chicago, il USA.

Maroudas AI. 1976. Balance between swelling pressure and collagen tension in normal and degenerate cartilage. *Nature* 260(5554):808-9.

Matzelle TR, Ivanov DA, Landwehr D, Heinrich LA, Herkt BC, Reichelt R, Kruse N. 2002. Micromechanical properties of "smart" gels: Studies by scanning force and scanning electron microscopy of pnipaam. *J. Phys. Chem. B* 106(11):2861 66.

McDevitt CA, Muir H. 1976. Biochemical changes in the cartilage of the knee in experimental and natural osteoarthritis in the dog. *J Bone Joint Surg Br* 58(1):94-101.

Mow VC, Kuei SC, Lai WM, Armstrong CG. 1980. Biphasic creep and stress relaxation of articular cartilage in compression? Theory and experiments. *J Biomech Eng* 102(1):73-84.

Oliver WC, Pharr GM. 1992. An improved technique for determining hardness and elastic modulus using load and displacement sensing indentation experiments. *Journal of Materials Research* vol.7, no.6; June 1992; p.1564 83.

Persch G, Born C, Utesch B. 1994. Nano-hardness investigations of thin films by an atomic force microscope. *Microelectronic Engineering* vol.24, no.1 4; March 1994; p.113 21.

Pharr GM, Oliver WC. 1992. Measurement of thin film mechanical properties using nanoindentation. *MRS Bulletin* vol.17, no.7; July 1992; p.28 33.

Pharr GM, Oliver WC, Brotzen FR. 1992. On the generality of the relationship among contact stiffness, contact area, and elastic modulus during indentation. *Journal of Materials Research* vol.7, no.3; March 1992; p.613 17.

Polisson R. 2001. Innovative therapies in osteoarthritis. *Curr Rheumatol Rep* 3(6):489-95.

Popko J, Mnich Z, Wasilewski A, Latosiewicz R. 1986. Topographic differences in the value of the 2 sec elastic modul in the cartilage tissue of the knee joint. *Beitr Orthop Traumatol* 33(10):506-9.

Radmacher M. 1997. Measuring the elastic properties of biological samples with the afm. *IEEE Eng Med Biol Mag* 16(2):47-57.

Radmacher M, Fritz M, Hansma PK. 1995. Imaging soft samples with the atomic force microscope: Gelatin in water and propanol. *Biophys J* 69(1):264-70.

Randall NX, Julia SC, Soro JM. 1998. Combining scanning force microscopy with nanoindentation for more complete characterisation of bulk and coated materials. *Surface and Coatings Technology* vol.108 109, no.1 3; 10 Oct. 1998; p.489 95.

Rho JY, Tsui TY, Pharr GM. 1997. Elastic properties of human cortical and trabecular lamellar bone measured by nanoindentation. *Biomaterials* 18(20):1325-30.

Ross R. 1986. The pathogenesis of atherosclerosis--an update. *N Engl J Med* 314(8):488-500.

Roth V, Mow VC. 1980. The intrinsic tensile behavior of the matrix of bovine articular cartilage and its variation with age. *J Bone Joint Surg Am* 62(7):1102-17.

Rotsch C, Jacobson K, Radmacher M. 1999. Dimensional and mechanical dynamics of active and stable edges in motile fibroblasts investigated by using atomic force microscopy. *Proc Natl Acad Sci U S A* 96(3):921-6.

Rotsch C, Radmacher M. 2000. Drug-induced changes of cytoskeletal structure and mechanics in fibroblasts: An atomic force microscopy study. *Biophysical Journal* vol.78, no.1, pt.1; Jan. 2000; p.520 35.

Shepherd DE, Seedhom BB. 1997. A technique for measuring the compressive modulus of articular cartilage under physiological loading rates with preliminary results. *Proc Inst Mech Eng [H]* 211(2):155-65.

Sneddon IN. 1965. The relation between load and penetration in the axisymmetric boussinesq problem for a punch of arbitrary profile. *Int. J. Engng Sci* 3:47–57.

Stolz M, Seidel J, Martin I, Raiteri R, Aebi U, Baschong W. 1999. Ex vivo measurement of the elasticity of extracellular matrix constituents by atomic force microscopy (afm). *Mol. Biol. Cell 10, 145a.*

Swanepoel MW, Smeathers JE, Adams LM. 1994. The stiffness of human apophyseal articular cartilage as an indicator of joint loading. *Proceedings of the Institution of Mechanical Engineers, Part H (Journal of Engineering in Medicine)* vol.208, no.H1; 1994; p.33 43.

Tkaczuk H. 1986. Human cartilage stiffness. In vivo studies. *Clin Orthop*(206):301-12.

Torii A, Sasaki M, Hane K, Okuma S. 1996. A method for determining the spring constant of cantilevers for atomic force microscopy. *Measurement Science & Technology* vol.7, no 2; p.179 84.

Turner CH, Rho J, Takano Y, Tsui TY, Pharr GM. 1999. The elastic properties of trabecular and cortical bone tissues are similar: Results from two microscopic measurement techniques. *Journal of Biomechanics* vol.32, no.4; April 1999; p.437 41.

Van den Berg WB, Van der Kraan PM, Scharstuhl A, Van Beuningen HM. 2001. Growth factors and cartilage repair. *Clin Orthop*(391 Suppl):S244-50.

VanLandingham MR, Dagastine RR, Eduljee RF, McCullough RL, Gillespie JW, Jr. 1999. Characterization of nanoscale property variations in polymer composite systems: Part 1 -- experimental results. *Composites Part A* vol.30, no.1;1999; p.75 83.

VanLandingham MR, McKnight SH, Palmese GR, Bogetti TA, Eduljee RF, Gillespie JW, Jr., Braint CL, Carter CB, Hall EL. 1997a. Characterization of interphase regions using atomic force microscopy. *Interfacial Engineering for Optimized Properties. Symposium. Mater. Res. Soc, Pittsburgh, PA, USA* xiv+510 pp.

VanLandingham MR, McKnight SH, Palmese GR, Eduljee RF, Gillespie JW, McCullough RL, Jr. 1997b. Relating elastic modulus to indentation response using atomic force microscopy. *Journal of Materials Science Letters* vol.16, no.2; 15 Jan. 1997; p.117 19.

Vawter DL. 1983. Poisson's ratio and incompressibility. *Transactions of the ASME. Journal of Biomechanical Engineering*. vol.105, no.2; p.194 5.

Vinckier A, Semenza G. 1993. Measuring elasticity of biological materials by atomic force microscopy. *FEBS Lett* 430(1-2):12-6.

Virmani R, Kolodgie FD, Burke AP, Farb A, Schwartz SM. 2000. Lessons from sudden coronary death: A comprehensive morphological classification scheme for atherosclerotic lesions. *Arterioscler Thromb Vasc Biol* 20(5):1262-75.

Walch M, Ziegler J, Groscurth P. 2000. Effect of streptolysin o on the microelasticity of human platelets analyzed by atomic force microscopy. *Ultramicroscopy* vol.82, no.14; Feb. 2000; p.259 67.

Weisenhorn AL, Kasas S, Solletti JM, Khorsandi M, Gotzos V, Romer DU, Lorenzi GP. 1993a. Deformation observed on soft surfaces with an afm. *Proceedings of the SPIE The International Society for Optical Engineering* vol.1855; 1993; p.26 34.

Weisenhorn AL, Khorsandi M, Kasas S, Gotzos V, Butt HJ. 1993b. Deformation and height anomaly of soft surfaces studied with an afm. *Nanotechnology* vol.4, no.2; April 1993; p.106 13.

Weisenhorn AL, Maivald P, Butt HJ, Hansma PK. 1992. Measuring adhesion, attraction, and repulsion between surfaces in liquids with an atomic force microscope. *Physical Review B (Condensed Matter)* vol.45, no.19; 15 May 1992; p.11226 32.

6. Summary and Outlook

6 Summary and outlook

6.1 There is no such thing like an ideal microscope

For a detailed understanding of biological tissues and proteins and their dynamical processes the 3D structures of the components involved must be known. Most of the structural data have been obtained through the combination of three major techniques: X-ray crystallography, NMR and TEM. These three methods enable the determination of the structure of biological macromolecules at near atomic resolution and each of those was developed over many years to perfection. Nevertheless each one has its advantage and limitations and all of them may be considered today as useful and complementary tools (Schabert and Engel 1995).

In addition to those established techniques, probably the most spectacular advances have been achieved with the AFM, which is the first imaging device allowing direct correlation between structural and functional states of biomolecules in their physiological environment over a range of scaling very much comparable to the capabilities of EM. Moreover, the AFM has the striking possibility to observe biological matter with high resolution in space, time and applied force and with a striking signal-to-noise ratio that typically allows to directly using unprocessed data.

Using time-lapse AFM, it is possible to monitor the structural and conformational changes with various biological processes such as the assembly/ disassembly mechanisms of proteins. The AFM tip can also be used to manipulate and control single molecules with forces in the piconewton range. Two interesting examples are the mechanical unfolding of proteins and the measurement of the actin-myosin interaction force.

Theoretically the AFM enables to image, probe and manipulate biomolecules in a fully native state at submolecular resolution. However, at the moment this is only feasible for reconstituted transmembrane proteins that are forming 2D crystals *in vitro*. Imaging of a huge variety of other interesting specimens, e.g. DNA, motor proteins, living cells or the sponge like nuclear pore complex, only reveal macromolecular or even a poorer resolution and protocols for investigating and analyzing other types of biological samples, e.g. connective tissues (cartilage, tendon, bone) or the plaque particles in the coronary arteries, so far are not worked out. In this doctoral thesis I refined or developed several new preparation protocols applicable for the investigation on a variety of biological or medical relevant samples:

In a first project we applied high resolution AFM imaging to the luminal and cytoplasmic face of the asymmetric unit membrane (AUM) of the urine bladder epithelium that forms 2D crystalline plaques *in vivo*. Those urothelial plaques are meant to be involved in a variety of pathological processes, like bladder cancer that ranges among the five most frequent cancer diseases. Moreover, the investigation of AUM in the AFM could offer a basic understanding of the plaque forming process at the innermost part of the bladder, which potentially might also give new insights into a wide variety of structural and dynamical changes occurring in a lipid membrane *in situ*.

In a second project we succeeded to establish a protocol for the robust immobilization of different assemblies of the water soluble protein actin, a 43-kDa protein that plays a fundamental role in muscle contraction, cytoskeletal processes and motility. We achieved high-resolution AFM images of the G- and F-actin arrays that hold promise for detailed structural analyses at the molecular level of morphological changes induced by chemical effectors. This project aims ultimately to trace the muscle-dynamics in its different conformational steps throughout the ATPase/ cross-bridge cycle and at the level of single molecules, i.e. to trace the mechanical interaction of the molecular motor myosin with actin filaments.

In a third project we developed new preparation and evaluation protocols that should enable us to directly measure the critical biomechanical parameters of soft biological tissue at the micrometer to nanometer scale. Therefore AFM imaging and indentation-based AFM have enabled us to trace alterations of the tissue architecture at all relevant scales. As a first clinically relevant sample we imaged and mechanically tested articular cartilage in its normal state and compared it to a disease state caused by osteoarthritis. These results are paving new vistas for monitoring disease processes at the scale they are actually occurring, i.e. at the cellular to molecular level. Elasticity measurements at different scales on native articular cartilage provided us with a better understanding of cartilage biomechanics and offer new possibilities in mapping cartilage mechanical properties, which will also include the viscoelastic properties in further measurements.

In a next step, individual building blocks were specifically removed out of the tissue architecture by enzyme action. Those digestion experiments helped us to model or mimic alterations caused by pathological degradation processes. At this stage sufficiently smooth samples for high resolution imaging can only be prepared from frozen samples by employing cryo-microtomy. For a refinement of the procedure a protocol has to be developed for combining high resolution imaging with the mechanical probing at the specific sites of interest. Of course the final goal would be that all preparation steps could be done under near physiological conditions.

Concerning clinically relevant applications, this work opens the possibility of an *in vivo* analysis of cartilage consistence in the knee or the investigation of plaque particles in the coronary arteries. This directly leads to the ultimate goal of *in situ* force mapping by a minimally invasive procedure, i.e. by incorporating the AFM into an arthroscope or into a heart catheter.

In summary: In the context of structural research in biology and medicine the AFM is a sensitive microscopical technique with exciting new possibilities to explore new areas of revealing interactions of molecules and merging them with those obtained in the related fields of biochemistry and genetics or by different techniques to gain a comprehensive understanding of cell function: motility, organelle dynamics, membrane transport, and regulation. Moreover, it might be very useful to integrate AFM and AFM-based techniques rather than separating the different techniques and disciplines. Structural, genetical and biochemical data might eventually be composed with the intermediate resolution of EM and AFM and atomic resolution achieved by X-ray crystallography and NMR. In a truly integrated approach the AFM should be complementary to – and not competing with – other microscopical techniques, diffraction methods and spectroscopies.

6.2 Further developments in instrumentation

The power of AFM is rooted in its unique capabilities of an extremely high dimensional resolution capability and its resolution in applying and/ or measuring forces that potentially allows the tracing of the fundamental biological processes of life, for example, the translocation of mRNA into protein by the ribosome, the production of molecular "fuel" (e.g., ATP) in mitochondria, and the translocation of ions and small molecules across membranes by channels and pumps. Further developments in sample preparation and instrumentation will open up new AFM capabilities in terms of high-resolution imaging, a better temporal resolution in time-lapse imaging, therefore leading to a real-time imaging and a more time efficient force-mapping and maybe a direct data processing.

A higher spatial resolution could be achieved by employing a more sensitive feedback system that requires lower loading forces in combination or in addition to novel and more efficient operational modes, like an improved and more sensitive tapping mode or even better, a real non-contact mode in liquid.

Currently new AFMs are designed that are specialized for faster recording of data (Ando et al. 2001; Viani et al. 1999). These instruments operate shorter cantilevers with low-noise characteristics that respond much faster than those currently in use. The new design allows much higher image speed for tapping mode in liquid and also drastically reduces the time for force mapping. Recently a scan rate of up to one frame per second and one to a few minutes for the force mapping have been achieved respectively. This is an important step to trace conformational changes of biological matter in their physiological states and studying the dynamic processes in real time. In combination with more specific software this eventually allows the recording frames at video speed in the future.

As stated in the introduction, AFM does not only provide the "eyes" for high resolution imaging but it also provides the "fingers" to measure and manipulate matter at the atomic and molecular level. This is of great relevance in the life sciences: Recently it has been demonstrated by dissecting DNA from a particular part of the chromosome that the probe can also be used as a nanoscalpel to dissect fragile biological samples (Thalhammer et al. 1997).

In this context, force-spectroscopy is another dedicated new methodology, which continuously is under development for investigation, the dynamical processes occurring during the unfolding of a biomolecule (Oesterhelt et al. 2000; Rief et al. 2000; Rief et al. 1997). It might be possible to determine forces generated by a biomolecule on the microsecond time scale. A faster and more sensitive force-spectroscopy based on AFM might allow studying biological processes with greater resolution in time and applied force.

By employing IT AFM the tip can be placed directly atop individual structural features to measure its biomechanical properties. In this doctoral thesis I have demonstrated that biomechanical information such as the elastic modulus can be strongly dependent on the experimental scale which is given by the size of the indenter. This could be especially interesting for putative clinical applications, such as obtaining clinical relevant information at fundamentally different levels of tissues architecture.

6.2.1 Probes

The attainable spatial resolution is directly related to the shape and sharpness of the scanning probe tip. The apex of commercially available tips typically has typical radii of curvature of some nanometers (Czajkowsky et al. 2000) and will improve in the future in terms of sharpness and in reduction of cantilever noise. There may be a practical advantage in using other tips grown *in situ* onto cantilevers or carbon nanotubes using an electron microscope. Both types of tips possess many unique properties that make them ideal AFM probes. Their high aspect ratio provides faithful imaging of deep trenches, while good resolution is retained due to their nanometer-scale diameter. These geometrical factors also lead to reduce tip-sample adhesion, which therefore might allow a gentler imaging.

New types of cantilevers might be more specific in terms of their physical or chemical functioning of the probe or on the other hand biochemically compatible for biomedical applications. Multifunctional cantilevers will provide the extension to a whole set of new experimental opportunities of monitoring possibly a wide range of multiple signals, like voltage, currents of ions or electrons and fluorescently labeled molecules (Engel et al. 1999).

Nanotubes are electrically conductive, which allow their use for the measurements of (surface-) potentials, and they can be modified at their ends with specific chemical or biological groups for high resolution functional imaging. Nanotubes could also be used as nanopipettes for drug delivery or as an electrical conductive tip for measuring local potentials, currents or trafficking of biomolecules across membranes.

Arrays of cantilevers (millipede) are under development that could be used for mechanically probing simultaneously neighboring regions of the specimen. This could allow mapping mechanical properties or imaging of larger regions within a short time or a more reliable diagnosis, i.e. different tissues or the plaques in the coronal arteries involved in heart diseases, all of them with an extremely high interest for medical research and treatment of diseases.

Combined AFM-SNOM (scanning near-field optical microscopy) - probe tips are potentially of great use and can be handled almost like the commonly used AFM probes. SNOM allows the detection of a conventional AFM height image and additionally an optical image with an improved optical resolution of more than one order of magnitude compared to conventional LM. SNOM therefore offers in addition to the topography also corresponding optical information of fluorescently labeled biological features beyond the diffraction limit of conventional light microscopy. One potential application might be the detection of the green fluorescent protein expressed by some cell strains. These tips can either be used as a detector to follow for example the specimen of green fluorescent proteins or as an effector to induce photoactive processes at the single molecule level.

One of our future projects is to detect the bidirectional trafficking through the nuclear pore complex by fluorescently labeled cargo. To achieve this we are developing a protocol to tightly seal the nuclear envelope of Xenopus oozytes over microfabricated pores. The goal is to measure in their complete functional state the transport rates of these nuclear gates at the level of single pores. In a comparison with genetically modified pores we aim to understand the regulation of cargoes between the nucleus and cytoplasm.

6.2.2 Putative applications of AFM-based techniques in medicine

The impacts of nano science in medically relevant applications foster the development of new devices and analytical tools for clinical practice. Due to the very high signal-to-noise ratio, AFM-based techniques offer the observation, probing and characterization of the chemical and mechanical properties of single molecules within a tissue in a physiologically relevant environment. Therefore pathological changes in human tissue can be registered and hopefully cured at an early stage of the disease progression. On the other hand by expanding our ability to characterize and control biological tissue in much more detail diagnostics and therapeutics could be revolutionized in terms of delivery of drugs in small amounts with a high resolution to the target.

The new possibilities opened by the AFM will also have an important impact for engineering and (quality-) control of surface properties of new biocompatible implants, tissue-engineered organs or novel biodegradable products that can be resorbed by the body after use. Progress in nanobiotechnology will promote the healing of natural tissue and will stimulate mimicking high-performance biocompatible nanosystems such as artificial active components or biological implants for organ and joint replacement. Thus new implants will be designed with nanoscale features that will replace degenerated, diseased or damaged tissues, e.g. arthritic cartilage or bone.

Since its invention the AFM has opened new avenues for a wide range of exciting applications ranging from basic structural research up to new developments for *in situ* applications in a clinical environment. However, diseases are often caused largely by damages either at the molecular or the cellular scale. For a local assessment today's surgical tools are simply too big. In the future we should get tools that are molecular, both in their size and their precision; and then we will be able to intervene directly at the level where the damage occurs and correct it. Ultimately the dream of Richard Feynman and Albert R. Hibbs might become true that once nanoscale machines can be injected into the bloodstream for dialysis or drug delivery.

6.3 References

Ando T, Kodera N, Takai E, Maruyama D, Saito K, Toda A. 2001. A high-speed atomic force microscope for studying biological macromolecules. *Proc Natl Acad Sci U S A* 98(22):12468-72.

Czajkowsky DM, Iwamoto H, Shao Z. 2000. Atomic force microscopy in structural biology: From the subcellular to the submolecular. *J Electron Microsc* 49(3):395-406.

Engel A, Lyubchenko Y, Muller D. 1999. Atomic force microscopy: A powerful tool to observe biomolecules at work. *Trends Cell Biol* 9(2):77-80.

Oesterhelt F, Oesterhelt D, Pfeiffer M, Engel A, Gaub HE, Muller DJ. 2000. Unfolding pathways of individual bacteriorhodopsins. *Science* 288(5463):143-6.

Rief M, Gautel M, Gaub HE. 2000. Unfolding forces of titin and fibronectin domains directly measured by AFM. *Adv Exp Med Biol* 481:129-36.

Rief M, Gautel M, Oesterhelt F, Fernandez JM, Gaub HE. 1997. Reversible unfolding of individual titin immunoglobulin domains by AFM. *Science* 276(5315):1109-12.

Schabert FA, Engel A. 1995. Atomic force microscopy of biological membranes: Current possibilities and prospects. *Forces in Scanning probe Methods*:607-614.

Thalhammer S, Stark RW, Muller S, Wienberg J, Heckl WM. 1997. The atomic force microscope as a new microdissecting tool for the generation of genetic probes. *J Struct Biol* 119(2):232-7.

Viani MB, Schaffer TE, Palcczi GT, Pietrasanta I, Smith BL, Thompson JB, Richter M, Rief M, Gaub HE, Plaxco KW et al. 1999. Fast imaging and fast force spectroscopy of single biopolymers with a new atomic force microscope designed for small cantilevers. *Review of Scientific Instruments. vol.70, no.11; Nov. 1999; p.4300 3.*

Acknowledgements

Acknowledgements

I want to gratefully acknowledge all who supported me during the time of this thesis.

Especially, I want to thank Prof. Dr. Ueli Aebi. After 5 years under Ueli's supervision I am sure that this was the best place for doing my PhD. Yes, it's true, without Ueli I certainly would have left science by now. I had numerous discussions with Ueli and am grateful that he shared many of his insights and knowledge with me. This fruitful time here at the M.E. Müller Institute let me almost forgot about my initial plans, i.e. to take my green card for starting a businessman career in the United States. In particular, I have appreciated the very high standard of equipment and science he provided here at this very special institute. In addition, I enjoy that Ueli involves me in science management by giving me the opportunity to participate and learn from a very interesting person and a brilliant scientist.

I thank Prof. Dr. Andreas Engel. The time I started my Ph.D. he was already famous for his AFM work on 2D protein crystals. His beautiful AFM images were a great inspiration and motivation for me to use the AFM in my way for working on biological matter. It is a pleasure but also a challenge to have with Andreas and Ueli such outstanding scientists at the same institute.

I thank Dr. Cora-Ann Schönenberger who is an excellent scientist with a clear scientific mind. Cora taught me the basics of biology. She has always been willing to help me through any difficulties with biology, especially at the beginning of my endeavor in the life sciences. She is the good heart in our lab and she supported me during the hard time when my mother died.

I thank Dr. Markus Dürrenberger. He is a very creative person who enriches the lab with his ideas, his generous support and his very positive attitude towards people. Markus has the knowledge and drive to find solutions for smaller or bigger difficulties in terms of equipment and new developments. Thank you Markus!

I thank Dr. Werner Baschong. With my measurements on cartilage tissue, I made the step from the world of biology directly into the world of medicine. Well, from my initial background as a physicist the world of medicine looks quite different! In this endeavor, Werner provided me with a new way of understanding. Werner usually is the first person for me to discuss "Gedankenexperimente" in terms of feasibility of new ideas and their putative potential in medicine.

Acknowledgements

I thank Markus Häner. He clearly impressed me about his skills in operating the transmission electron microscope – pure perfection! It was a great pleasure to learn from him. Moreover, it was a great pleasure to share some time with such a nice person and colleague. He left this world too early!

I thank Clemens Möller. I enjoyed our discussions about girls, physics, biology, politics and many other subjects. I spent with him the most time in and out of the lab.

I thank Dr. Jochen Köser, our "Kiwies" from New Zealand Dr. Claire Goldsbury and Janelle Green, Dr. Bernd Feja, Dr. Daniel Stoffler, Dr. Birthe Fahrenkrog, Dr. Anna Mandinova, Melanie Börries, Daphna Atar, Dr. Veronique Brault, Alumalla-Venkateshwar Reddy, Dr. Herve Remigy, Dr. Dimitrios Fotiatis, Dr. Henning Stahlberg, Dr. Daniel Müller, Dr. Lorenz Hasler and all the others from the Aebi lab and the Engel lab that are nice colleagues and who made my life at this place comfortable and pleasant.

Special thanks to Ursula Sauders and Rosemarie Sütterlin who helped me with their technical know how in sample preparations.

Special thanks to Liselotte Walti, our secretary, for taking care of the administrative paper work.

Special thanks also for our technical crew, especially Robert Wyss, our mechanical engineer, and Robert Häring, our electronical engineer, who are taking care for the microscopes, computes and all the other machines and provide the very high standard of the lab. Many thanks for realizing some extra developments of equipment that was not available from the shelf.

And many thanks to other people not mentioned explicitly.

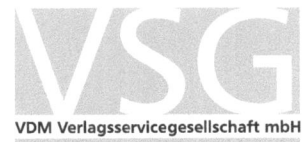

Die VDM Verlagsservicegesellschaft sucht für wissenschaftliche Verlage abgeschlossene und herausragende

Dissertationen, Habilitationen, Diplomarbeiten, Master Theses, Magisterarbeiten usw.

für die kostenlose Publikation als Fachbuch.

Sie verfügen über eine Arbeit, die hohen inhaltlichen und formalen Ansprüchen genügt, und haben Interesse an einer honorarvergüteten Publikation?

Dann senden Sie bitte erste Informationen über sich und Ihre Arbeit per Email an *info@vdm-vsg.de*.

Sie erhalten kurzfristig unser Feedback!

VDM Verlagsservicegesellschaft mbH
Dudweiler Landstr. 99
D - 66123 Saarbrücken
Telefon +49 681 3720 174
Fax   +49 681 3720 1749

www.vdm-vsg.de

Die VDM Verlagsservicegesellschaft mbH vertritt

 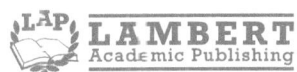 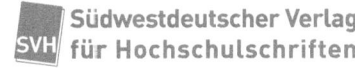

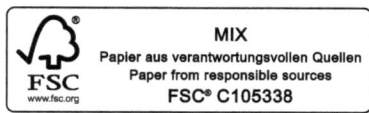

Printed by Books on Demand GmbH, Norderstedt / Germany